Recent Concept on Repeat Breeding in Dairy Cattle

Recent Concept on Repeat Breeding in Dairy Cattle

Dr. Dibyajyoti Talukdar
B.V.Sc. & A.H., M.V.Sc., Ph.D.
Teaching Associate
Department of Animal Reproduction, Gynaecology & Obstetrics
College of Veterinary Sciences & Animal Husbandry
Central Agricultural University, Selesih, Aizawl, Mizoram

Dr. Papori Talukdar
B.V.Sc. & A.H., M.V.Sc., Ph.D.
Assistant Professor
Department of Animal Nutrition
Khalsa College of Veterinary & Animal Sciences
Khalsa University, Amritsar, Punjab

SSPH

SATISH SERIAL PUBLISHING HOUSE
403, Express Tower, Commercial Complex
Azadpur, Delhi-110033 (India)
Phone : 011-27672852, Fax : 91-11-27672046
e-mail : info@satishserial.com, hkjain1975@yahoo.com
Website : www.satishserial.com

Published by :

SATISH SERIAL PUBLISHING HOUSE

403, Express Tower, Commercial Complex, Azadpur, Delhi-110033 (INDIA)
Phone : 011-27672852 Fax : 91-11-27672046
E-mail : info@satishserial.com, hkjain1975@yahoo.com

ISBN 978-93-86200-10-5

Composed, Designed & Printed in India

Dedicated to my beloved

respected teacher

Dr. K.C. Nath

Foreword

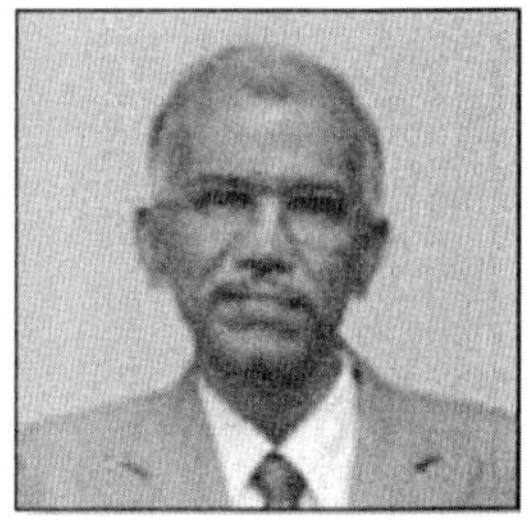

The success of dairy economics lies in ensuring proper and optimal reproductive rhythm of each individual cow in the herd, within normal physiological range. Any deviation or prolongation in the breeding rhythm results in a progressive economic loss due to widening of dry period, reduced calving and lactations during the life spans of the animal. Thus fertility of milch animals plays a vital role in dairy economics. It was estimated that even in well managed herds, the incidence of infertility ranged from 15 to 20 per cent, majority of which was due to repeat breeding syndrome. The problem of repeat breeding in crossbred cows has been noticed as a major reproductive problem in dairy cattle that affects fertility. It has multi-factorial etiology. It was estimated that even in well managed herds, the incidence of infertility ranged from 15 to 20 per cent, majority of which was due to repeat breeding syndrome. The problem of repeat breeding in crossbred cows has been noticed as a major reproductive problem in dairy cattle that affects fertility. The etiological factors are infectious, inflammatory processes, nutritional deficiencies, managemental error, ovulatory disturbances etc. Hence it has multi-factorial etiology, before going to therapeutic management one should have thorough knowledge about the different causes, its diagnostic procedure and its accurate treatment. The monograph provides in depth information on repeat breeding, different causes of repeat breeding, blood biochemical and hormonal changes in repeat breeder cow, the detail diagnostic methods and efficacy of different treatment protocols for repeat breeding in dairy cattle and its impact on dairy industry. Authors have done excellent job to collect the valuable informations on repeat breeding and share own experience in the practical fields and bring them together in this monograph for which they deserve all appreciation. I hope the monograph shall certainly be of immense value to the scientists, students, field Veterinarians and all other personnel concerned with repeat breeding in dairy cattle.

Date: 14.03.2017

D. Kathiresan
Dean
College of Veterinary Sciences & Animal Husbandry
Central Agricultural University
Selesih, Aizawl- 796014, Mizoram

Preface

Repeat breeding syndrome (RBS) is a serious problem in dairy industry leading to economic loss due to more inseminations, increased calving interval and culling rates. It was estimated that even in well managed herds, the incidence of infertility ranged from 15 to 20 per cent, majority of which was due to repeat breeding syndrome. The problem of repeat breeding in crossbred cows has been noticed as a major reproductive problem affecting both the small and large scale milch herds. If we see the economics, livestock farming is an integral subsidiary of Indian agriculture and dairying has become an important secondary source of income for millions of rural households engaged in agriculture. While the success of dairy economics lies in ensuring proper and optimal reproductive rhythm of each individual cow in the herd, within normal physiological range. Any deviation or prolongation in the breeding rhythm results in a progressive economic loss due to widening of dry period, reduced calving and lactations during the life spans of the dairy cattle. RBS is a multi factorial problem involving a number of extrinsic factors as well as intrinsic factors coupled to the individual animal. Before going to treatment, one should have the proper idea and diagnostic skill about the cause involve for the repeat breeding. If we know the actual cause responsible for this syndrome then we will achieve 100 per cent success rate. Here in this book, we will try to give you the complete idea regarding various causes of repeat breeding, the new diagnostic up to date methods and the current therapeutic management of the repeat breeding so that the incidence can be minimized. We hope, this book will be useful to the students, Scientist as well as the field Veterinarians and all other personnel concerned with repeat breeding for better knowledge and further research.

Dibyajyoti Talukdar
Papori Talukdar

Acknowledgement

We both the authors of the book entitled "Recent Concept on Repeat Breeding in Dairy Cattle" express our sincere thanks to Prof. (Dr) D. Kathiresan, Dean, College of Veterinary Sciences & Animal Husbandry, Central Agricultural University, Selesih, Aizawl, Mizoram for his moral support in preparation of this manuscript and sparing his valuable time in writing the foreword message for the book.

We express our sincere gratitude to Dr. F.A. Ahmed, Dr. K. Lalrintlunga, Dr. R. S. Arya, and Dr. G. Kalita for their constructive suggestions and help throughout the preparation of this manuscript.

We shall remain indebted to Dr. Kalyan Sarma for his consistent and invaluable inspirations, prolific and introspective guidance with constructive suggestions, deliberative discussions and active persuasion throughout the period of preparation of the book.

We also take this opportunity to extend our sincere thanks to all our teachers specially Dr. K.C. Nath, Dr. B.C. Deka, Dr. K.Ahmed, Dr. K.K. Bonia, Dr. J.Goswami, Dr. P.M. Barua, Dr. K.C. Deka, Dr. A. Sarma, Dr. D. Kalita, Dr. B. Saikia, Dr. S.S. Kundu, Dr. G. Mondal etc. who created interest for the subject in our mind and soul. Their constant guidance and encouragement enabled us to prepare this book.

We feel very proud to express our reverence and gratefulness to our parents for their affection, constant support, encouragement and blessings which enabled us to complete this book. They have always been the source of inspiration along the way in pursuing this endeavour.

Our sincere thanks are also due to the publishing agency Satish Serial Publishing House, Delhi, India for designing and publishing the book and making it a reality.

We look forward to receive constructive suggestions, if any, from the readers which will help us in improving the quality of the book in its future edition.

Dibyajyoti Talukdar
Papori Talukdar

Abbreviations

%	:	Percentage
<	:	Less than
>	:	Greater than
AI	:	Artificial insemination
ALP	:	Alkaline phosphatase
ALT	:	Alanine aminotransferase
AST	:	Aspartate aminotransferase
CAMP	:	Cyclic adenosine monophosphate
CL	:	Corpus luteum
cm	:	centimeter
CPK	:	Creatine phosphokinase
dL	:	Deciliter
e.g.	:	For example
ET	:	Embryo transfer
etc.	:	Et Cetera (and so on)
FAS	:	Foreign Agricultural Service
FSH	:	Follicle stimulating hormone
gm	:	Gram
GoI	:	Govt. of India
hrs	:	hours
i.e.	:	That is
IM	:	Intramuscular
IU	:	International Unit
IV	:	Intravenous
IVF	:	In vitro fertilization
IVM	:	In vitro maturation
L	:	Litre
LDH	:	Lactic dehydrogenase

LH	:	Luteinizing hormone
mg	:	Milligram
Min	:	Minute
ml	:	Millilitre
mm	:	Millimeter
mmol	:	millimole
ng	:	Nanogram
°C	:	Degree Celsius
pg	:	picogram
SDH	:	Sorbitol dehydrogenase
U	:	Unit
USDA	:	United States Department of Agriculture
viz.	:	Namely
vs	:	Versus
w/v	:	Weight by volume
w/w	:	Weight by weight
μl	:	Microlitre

Contents

Chapter-1

Repeat Breeding Syndrome in Cattle and its Impact on Dairy Industry

Successful fertilisation is the result of well-timed sperm-oocyte interactions. Time of insemination and proper sperm transport to the site of fertilization, within the functional life span of the oocyte, is major prerequisites. In cattle, Repeat breeding syndrome (RBS) is a condition in which dairy animal have a regular oestrous cycle and appears normal on superficial clinical examination but fail to become pregnant following three or more breeding (Barlett *et al.*, 1986). It is a serious problem in dairy industry leading to economic loss due to more inseminations, increased calving interval and culling rates (Lafi *et al.*, 1992). It was estimated that even in well managed herds, the incidence of infertility ranged from 15 to 20 per cent, majority of which was due to repeat breeding syndrome. The problem of repeat breeding in crossbred cows has been noticed as a major reproductive problem affecting both the small and large scale milch herds.

RBS is a multi factorial problem involving a number of extrinsic factors as well as intrinsic factors coupled to the individual animal (Gustafsson and Emanuelson, 2002). The causes in broad sense can be divided into two categories, fertilization failure and early embryonic death (Amiridis *et al.*, 2009). In a study, Saxena (2004) reported the incidence of repeat breeding to be varied from 5.50 to 33.33% in cattle and from 6.00 to 30.00% in buffalo. The variability in the incidence may be due to heterogeneity of cause and effect of locality and season (Ali *et al.*, 2009). Failure of ovulation is one of the important causes of repeat breeding in cattle occurring in widely varying frequencies of

22.50 to 39.00 per cent as reported from India as well as from abroad (Van Rensburg and De Vos, 1962; Mehta *et al.*, 1986; Deka, 1994; Das, 2002). According to Morrow (1969) ovulation failure occurred in 13.2 per cent on their first standing oestrus and in 1.9 per cent on their second oestrus. The occurrence of anovulation was greater at first oestrus than at subsequent oestrus periods. It had been stated that failure of ovulation was due to a failure or insufficient release of luteinizing hormone (LH) from the anterior pituitary gland and associated with nutritional, hereditary and stress or work factors (Roberts, 1971). Poor semen quality or faulty AI techniques is considered as a major managemental factors in cattle which causes repeat breeding. Therefore the factors responsible for this malady is multiple viz. anatomical, hormonal, managemental and infectious and it may vary from herd to herd, animal to animal and oestrus to oestrus.

If we see the economics, livestock farming is an integral subsidiary of Indian agriculture. India earned the reputation of world's largest producer of milk with an annual production of 146.3 million tonne which is 18.5 % of world production (2014-15). This has been achieved at the cost of providing shelter to a huge component around 37.28% (190.90 million numbers as per the 19th Livestock census- 2012, GoI) of the total livestock population in India and 31.05% of world's cattle population (FAS/ USDA, 2016). The per capita availability of milk in India has increased from 176 grams per day in 1990-91 to 322 grams per day by 2014-15 (Economic survey 2015-16, presented by the Union Finance Minister, India). It is more than the world average of 294 grams per day during 2013. This signifies a continued growth in availability of milk and milk products for the growing population. Dairying has become an important secondary source of income for millions of rural households engaged in agriculture. While the success of dairy economics lies in ensuring proper and optimal reproductive rhythm of each individual cow in the herd, within normal physiological range. Any deviation or prolongation in the breeding rhythm results in a progressive economic loss due to widening of dry period, reduced calving and lactations during the life spans of the dairy cattle (Figure 1). Thus fertility of milch animals plays a vital role in dairy economics. It has been estimated that even in well managed herds, the incidence of infertility ranged from 15 to 20 per cent, majority of which was due to repeat breeding syndrome. The problem of repeat breeding in crossbred cows has been noticed as a major reproductive problem affecting both the small and large scale milch herds.

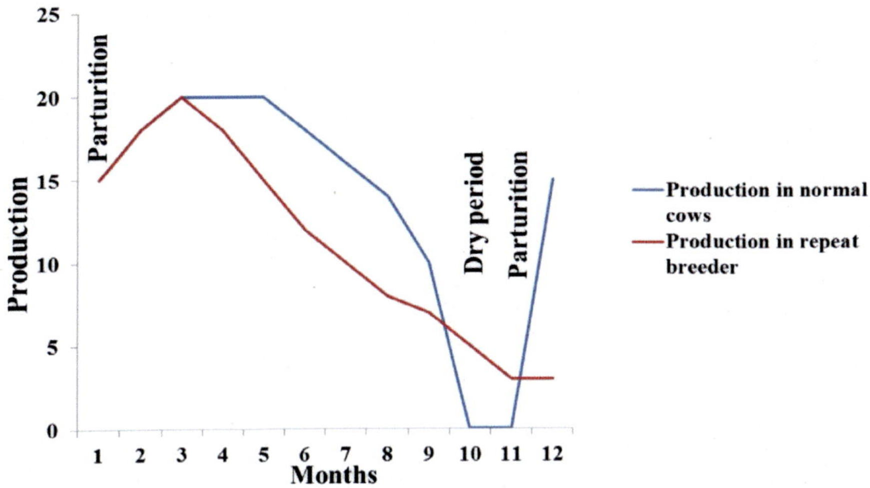

Figure 1. Milk production in normal cyclic and repeat breeder cow in one year, in where the repeat breeder cow having constant declining trend with long inter calving periods

To obtain a high reproductive efficiency in dairy cattle, it is necessary to get a calving interval of 365 days and an overall calving rate of 95% (Duffy *et al.*, 2004). The dairy cows should get pregnant around day 85 after calving. But in reality, it is not seen even in well managed herds. Studies carried out in US earlier; indicated that only between 50-70% of cows reach this goal. The production system presents notable differences with respect to reproductive indexes. Under intensive farming system, dairy cows the first parturition occurs at 28 months old. The preovulatory follicle size is correlated with the fertility of the animal, and it has been postulated that the implementation of good management practice helps to optimize the size of the ovulatory follicle which could improve the fertility (Duffy *et al.*, 2004). For getting good reproductive results it is recommended to select those animals that:

- Calved one alive and healthy calf per year.
- Get pregnant at three months after post partum.
- Have a good maternal condition during gestation and after gestation.
- Yields maximum during lactation.
- Free from any kind of reproductive disorder.

❑❑❑

Chapter-2

Various Etiological Factors Causing Repeat Breeding Syndrome

Repeat breeding is a serious infertility problem which reduces the productivity and economic efficiency of dairy cattle. Most of the repeat breeders are not sterile; rather they suffer from lowered fertility. Therefore a careful evaluation is warranted to define the most probable reason for the failure to conceive or failure to maintain pregnancy. This type of study also provided useful insight into risk factors associated with repeat breeding in dairy cows.

The author investigated 246 repeat breeder cows of three genetic groups (Holstein- Friesian crossbred, Jersey crossbred and local indigenous cows of Assam, India) managed in private farms located at Kamrup district of Assam, India during 2014-15. All the animals were maintained under stall-fed conditions with usual management practice and it categorized under five categories according to causes based on clinical findings *viz.*, anovulation, delayed ovulation, normal ovulation, uterine infection and genital anatomical abnormalities which occurring in the percentage of 34.95, 32.52, 8.13, 21.95 and 2.43 respectively (Figure 2). These findings indicated that ovulatory disturbances were the common cause of repeat breeding in cows accounting for more than 50 per cent of the cows reported to be repeat breeder. This discrepancy in the incidence of ovulatory disturbances might be due to variation in genetic makeup of the animal, level of nutrition and degree of stress (Roberts, 1971). The percentage of repeat breeder cow with normal ovulation was due to subclinical endometritis which might be the major contributor in causing repeat breeding in cattle under such circumstances (Noakes *et al.,* 2001). The percentage of repeat breeder cow that had uterine infection was 21.95 per cent (Talukdar *et al.,* 2016). The congenital or acquired anomalies of the genital canal were reported to be the infrequent cause for repeat breeding. These defects included principally the anomalies or segmental aplasia of oviduct, uterus, cervix and vagina, kinked cervix. The kinked cervix or hardness of cervix may appear due to trauma or lacerations during calving and AI followed by infection and fibrosis. The incidence of cervicitis varied from 0.9-5.52% in cattle (Amiridis *et al.,* 2009; Talukdar *et al.,* 2016) and 0.5-2 % in Indian buffalo (Kumar *et al.,* 1988). The another important anatomical anomaly *i.e.* ovaro-bursal adhesions (OBA) develop between ovary and ovarian bursa as a result of faulty handling of ovary, intrauterine infusion of irritating drugs in large volume under pressure and due to infections. The incidence of OBA has been reported earlier as 0.29-1.8 % in cattle (Kumar and Agarwal, 1986). This defects and anomalies of genital tract largely caused failure of fertilization by preventing the union of the sperm cell and the ovum (Roberts, 1971).

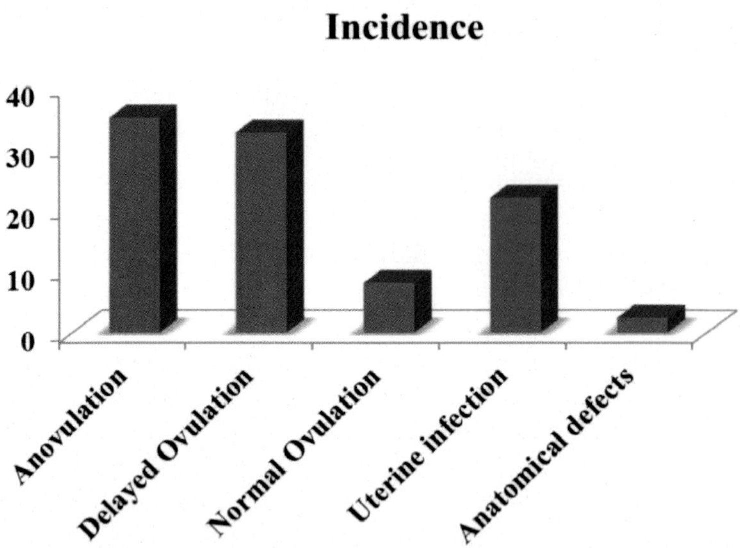

Figure 2. Incidences of different causes of repeat breeding in dairy cows on the basis of clinical findings (Talukdar *et al.*, 2016)

Early embryonic mortality is also considered as a reason for repeat breeding. Under normal physiological situations, low progesterone concentrations during estrus relate to increased tubal spontaneous contractility, whereas a decrease in tubal spontaneous contractility is related to increasing progesterone concentrations during the luteal phase have indicated that tubal function (in terms of gamete transport) during estrus could be altered by manipulating steroid hormone concentrations (Singh *et al.*, 2005). It is possible that the suprabasal progesterone concentrations present in repeat breeder cattle during estrus reduced tubal contractility, resulting in an impaired or delayed sperm transport from the sperm reservoir to the site of fertilization. The delay in sperm transport may contribute to substantial sperm death due to membrane and acrosome disruption, thus impairing fertilization. This delay could also lead to polyspermy by the ageing of the oocytes before they encounter the spermatozoa (Albihn, 1991). Then, the resulting zygotes would have poor developing capacity and would eventually undergo early embryonic mortality. The heifer would subsequently return to estrus. In addition, in vitro exposure of bovine spermatozoa to uterine lavage from repeat-breeding cows adversely affects sperm motility by lowering their ability to consume oxygen. This altered protein synthesis and secretions from the uterine tube of the cow is due to persistent dominant follicles (Singh *et al.*, 2005). Therefore, it appears that the tubal environment in repeat breeder is not favorable for maintaining the optimal fertilizing ability of spermatozoa.

However, among the breeds the highest incidence of repeat breeding was recorded in Holstein- Friesian crossbred (57.72%) than Jersey crossbred (35.77%) and lowest incidence recorded in local indigenous cattle (6.61%) by Talukdar *et al.* (2016). On the basis of clinical examination the percentage of anovulation, delayed ovulation, normal ovulation, uterine infection and genital anatomical abnormalities occurring in Holstein- Friesian crossbred was 36.61, 36.61, 7.04, 15.49 and 4.22 respectively. In Jersey crossbred the percentage of anovulation, delayed ovulation, normal ovulation and uterine infection was 38.63, 27.27, 4.54 and 29.54 respectively; while there was no any genital anatomical abnormality recorded in repeat breeder Jersey crossbred cattle. The corresponding figure in local indigenous cow that had delayed ovulation, normal ovulation and uterine infection was 25.00, 37.50 and 37.50 respectively, while there was no any genital anatomical abnormality and anovulation recorded in repeat breeder local cow. These findings indicated that ovulatory disturbances was the common cause of repeat breeding in cows accounting for more than 50 per cent of the cows recorded to be repeat breeder in both Holstein-Friesian and Jersey crossbred which is might be due to prolonged basal progesterone after oestrus (Perez-Marin and Espana, 2007). The LH release pattern is modified and follicle does not get the stimulus for ovulation to occur. The follicle continues growing and releases estradiol, which induces the formation of persistent follicles and delayed ovulation. Also, defective follicle recruitment during the middle- and late-luteal phases has been suggested as a cause of anovulation. An abnormal hormone environment may promote continuous development in the dominant follicle, impairing follicular function and oocyte quality, and thus reducing fertility (Stock and Fortune, 1993). Irregular and delayed ovulations have been associated with asynchrony between oestrus and ovulation, asynchrony of LH peak and ovulation, or incapacity for LH release (Duchens *et al.*, 1995). The LH peak characteristics are altered in repeat breeder and oestrous signs are less intense than in normal cows. However the repeat breeder with normal ovulation and uterine infection were recorded in higher frequency in local cattle.

Parity wise, the overall incidence of repeat breeding in respect of heifer, 1st, 2nd, 3rd, 4th, 5th and above lactating cow of Holstein- Friesian crossbred were 15.49, 11.26, 19.71, 30.98, 11.26 and 11.26 per cent respectively (Figure 3); in Jersey crossbred the corresponding percentage were 11.36, 9.09, 13.63, 25.00, 18.18 and 22.72 per cent respectively. While in local indigenous cattle repeat breeding recorded in heifer and 3rd lactating cow and percentage of incidence was 75.00 and 25.00 respectively as reported by Talukdar *et al.* (2016). These findings indicated that the highest incidence of repeat breeding recorded in 3rd parity cow of Holstein and Jersey crossbreds except local cow in which the incidence was highest in heifer. The main cause recorded as ovulatory disturbance of the animal. The incidence of repeat breeding was found higher in 3rd parity cow of Holstein-Friesian and Jersey crossbreds which are might be due to maximum milk production that causes lactational stress and hormonal imbalance. In contrast to these findings, Mitiku *et al.* (2012) reported that the prevalence of repeat breeders was highest in the seventh parity (50%) and lowest in the first parity (3.12%) and they also stated that as parity increased risk of repeat breeders was also increased. It has been widely reported that age impacts negatively on fertility, and higher repeat breeding rates have been described in old cows (Hewett, 1968). It is attributed to alterations in hypothalamic or pituitary hormonal levels or to inability of the ovary response (Bullman and Lamming,

1978). It has also been demonstrated the relationship between old age and low oocytes viability, what explains the fertility decline (Hewett, 1968). Studies in repeat breeding showed that age and breed affect the FSH and LH levels. It is supported that fertility in dairy cattle improves after the 1st or 2nd parturition, and decreases from the 4th or 5th, but it should be taken into account the time required for uterine involution or problems associated to puerperium (Shrestha *et al.*, 2004). While in local cattle the incidence of repeat breeding found higher in heifer which is might be due to inseminating at puberty period on the first sign of oestrus and hormonal secretion (Mitiku *et al.*, 2012).

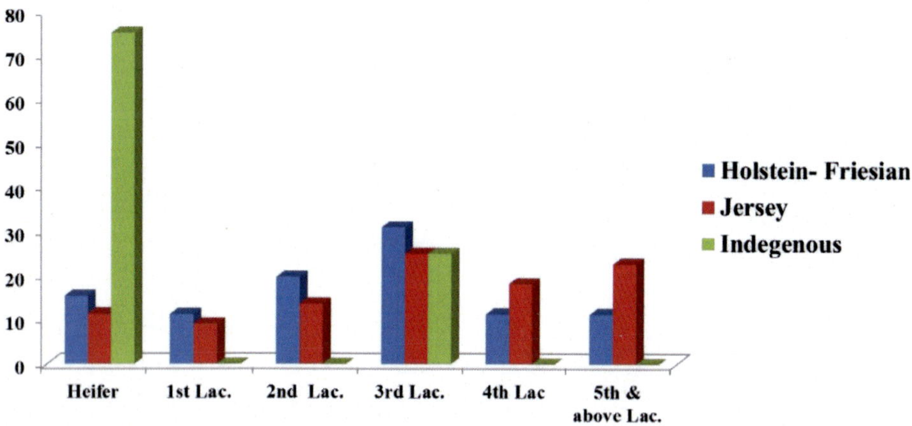

Figure 3. Incidence of repeat breeding in three different genetic grouped cows in respect of parities (Talukdar *et al.*, 2016)

Other Causes of Repeat Breeding

Repeat breeding as it discuss, is a serious problem and the first step in correcting it is to diagnose its cause or causes. Further this can be a difficult task since many factors can, and frequently do, contribute to a failure to conceive or maintain pregnancy. Other than individual cow problem it may be a herd problem or managemental failure. The herd problems are by far the most common, and those most often causing repeat breeding include:

Inadequate oestrus detection, resulting in improper timing of insemination in relation to the onset of standing estrus which may lead to repeat breeing syndrome. These cows being inseminated that have either early or late oestrus. The deposition of semen is closely related with the detection of oestrus and with all those factors that may affect the preovulatory LH. The cows mounting over the other cow are recognized as signs of the cow heat. This behaviour could last between 13-17 hr on average, and ovulation will take place approximately 30 hr after starting the heat. The semen is deposited in the female tract as close as possible to that time should be ensured. The morning/evening or AM/PM rule is the most common practice in dairy cattle farms: it consists of making insemination at morning if the cow was in heat the previous evening, or being inseminated in the afternoon if heat was detected in the morning. If the clinician palpates the ovaries before insemination and make sure that the follicle texture is far to ovulation, in this case double insemination is recommended separated by 12 hours.

The Bull factor and insemination techniques include:

a) Inadequate semen quality
b) Insufficient numbers of sperm
c) Infertile bull
d) Aging of sperm

The bull and its sperm quality must also be taken into account when repeat breeding causes are evaluated. It is essential to evaluate the sperm fertilizing ability in both natural mating and AI. Frozen semen straws should be carefully stored and managed. Repeat breeding could be linked to the above mentioned bull factors, in which oestrus is repeated and interestrus interval has normal duration.

The fertility of the bull should be optimum (either natural breeding or AI) to achieve high pregnancy rate and normal calving interval. The frozen semen doses are packed with 15-25 million of motile sperm prefreezing, because around 50% of spermatozoa recover motility after thawing. However, semen doses may fulfil all requirements; the donors of sperm should have erratic fertility. Therefore, strict selection of semen donors based on the semen quality after thawing and sexual behaviour, among other variables, has reduced defects in bulls used for the creation of frozen semen banks. At natural breeding also, it is essential to assess the reproductive performance of the bulls at least twice a year, carrying out semen assessment (macroscopic and microscopic) and physical evaluations. It is also mandatory to evaluate libido and the sexual behavioural pattern for mating to diagnose reproductive failures in bulls. On the other hand, maintenance of an appropriate male: female ratio for mating also advisable.

Summary

Repeat breeding is a serious infertility problem which reduces the productivity and economic efficiency of dairy cattle. Most of the repeat breeders are not sterile; rather they suffer from lowered fertility. Therefore a careful evaluation is warranted to define the most probable reason for the failure to conception or failure to maintain pregnancy. To correct the problem most successfully all parties should be involved in the reproductive management program, namely, the producer, inseminator and veterinarian, need to evaluate the problem and review the herd records together. This move towards the most rewarding since it helps to identify the number of factors, which alone may be minor, but collectively result in a herd problem. Inadequate oestrus detection is the most frequent cause of repeat breeding. So while diagnosing the cause of a repeat breeding, the oestrus detection program should always be thoroughly evaluated. When oestrus detection is faulty, standing oestrus is less likely to be observed and more cows are inseminated on the basis of signs other than standing oestrus. This results in inaccurate timing of insemination, which in turn results conception failure. If the herd owner undergoes natural service, then a thorough breeding soundness examination of the bull is indicated. This should include a complete diagnostic workup to identify any contributing physical factors or infectious agents. Sometimes the contributing factors are not willingly apparent and only become evident after all members of the management team have had to work together for betterment of the result.

❏❏❏

Chapter-3

Minerals and its Effect on Repeat Breeder Dairy Cattle

Appropriate management of dairy herd should be intended to optimize the production of the highest quality product and minimizing any adverse effects on the health and welfare of the animals (Harmon, 1998). In dairy cattle, we should give more emphasis on adequate nutrition and adequate mammary health of the animal so as to produce more and wholesome milk. Recent data indicate that the micro nutrient will enhance the production of good quality milk. The potential for minerals to play a significant role in herd fertility is indisputable. Due to high production and deficient feeding the productive animals are most commonly suffered with the nutritional deficiencies which ultimately leading to reduced reproductive performance. The minerals plays crucial role for growth and reproduction and are involved in a large number of digestive, physiological and biosynthetic processes within the body (Close, 1998). The most noticeable function is as constituents of body organs and tissues and to provide fundamental support. In addition, they act as electrolytes, as constituents of body fluids and as catalysts in both enzyme and hormone systems. Therefore they fulfill several important functions for the upkeep of animal growth and reproduction as well as health status (Underwood, 1981).

The mineral elements are categorized into major or macro minerals (calcium, phosphorous, potassium, sodium, chlorine, sulphur and magnesium) and trace or micro minerals (iron, iodine, copper, manganese, zinc, cobalt, molybdenum and selenium). The minerals that influence reproduction of the animal are generally found within the trace element group, although deficiencies of calcium and phosphorus can also affect fertility. Organic minerals have a positive role in resumption of follicular growth and fertility of the female animal. The usage of organic compared with inorganic forms, has been shown to enrich the survival rate and to increase fertilization rate (Lindemann, 1996). Organic minerals have several positive effects in ruminant and monogastric animals. There are still noticeable variances among chelated minerals, mineral proteins and other organic minerals complexes. Proteinated minerals perhaps improve reproduction of the female animal through increased fertilization, lower embryo mortality, improved uterine environment and/or increased intensity of estrus behavior. The importance of these minerals in reproductive performance of dairy cattle is given below.

Phosphorus (P)

There has been much argument on phosphorus supplementation and its effects on female reproductive function (Elrod and Butler, 1993). Deficiency of phosphorus may lead to decreased fertility rate, decreased ovarian activity, irregular oestrous cycles, increased occurrence of cystic ovaries, delayed sexual maturity and low conception rates have been reported (Cromwell, 1997). Heifers received only 70-80% of their phosphorus requirements showed impaired fertility (3.7 services per conception). Services per conception were reduced to 1.3 after adequate phosphorus was supplemented (Dunn and Moss, 1992). Increasing phosphorus supplementation from 0.4% to 0.6% of the ration had no effect on days to first oestrus or services per conception in another experiment. Nevertheless, in some instances, responses have been reported in the field when phosphorus supplementation was increased to 0.5% or 0.6%. The reason for these differences in response is unclear, but may be related to the availability of the phosphorus that is added to the ration or the actual amount of phosphorus consumed. An amount of 0.45 to 0.50 per cent phosphorus on dry matter basis should be provided to high producing cows (Schweigert and Zucker, 1988).

Calcium (Ca)

The ratios of Calcium and Phosphorus between 1.5:1 and 2.5:1 for lactating cows should not effect on reproduction. Sufficient amounts of calcium should always be provided to milking cows to exploit production and minimize health problems. One of the functions of calcium is to allow the muscle contraction. Reduction in muscle contractility will lead to a decrease in dry matter intake (DMI) as rumen function decreases, leading to severe Negative energy balance (NEB) which may increase in fat mobilization and as a result it may lead to fatty liver syndrome and ketosis. Uterine tonicity will also be adversely affected with cows experiencing prolonged calving and retained placenta. Uterine involution is not proper and it may impair fertility. Optimum levels of calcium and phosphorus should be provided to dry cows in order to decrease the occurrence of milk fever. The ration containing 0.75 to 0.80 per cent calcium on dry matter basis should be provided to high producing dairy animals (Schweigert and Zucker, 1988).

Selenium (Se)

Selenium has a significant role on normal spermatogenesis and largely as a component of seleno-proteins phospholipid hydroperoxide glutathione peroxidase (PHGPx/GPX4) and Seleno-protein V. Most of the selenium found in the testis is associated with PHGPx/GPX4. It serves as a powerful antioxidant defending cells from oxidative stress. PHGPx also appears to be involved as a structural protein to provide normal sperm motility (Hemler and Lands, 1980). It has also been reported that this protein is necessary for normal chromatin condensation and subsequent normal spermatozoa head formation. Both deficiency and excessive selenium have been proven to be detrimental to normal spermatogenesis (Wiltbank *et al.,* 2007). Marginally selenium deficient animals will abort, or calves will be weak and unable to stand or suckle. Adequate level of selenium supplementation may reduces the incidence of retained placentas, cystic ovaries, mastitis and metritis (Patterson *et al.,* 2003). In addition, cattle that maintain adequate blood selenium levels have reduced incidence of abortions, still births and peri-parturient recumbency (Pradhan and Nakaghosi, 2003). Chronic selenium toxicity causes lameness, sore feet, deformed claws and loss of hairs from tail. In pregnant animals, selenium toxicity will produce abortions, stillbirth and weak and lethargic calves as selenium accumulate in the foetus at the expense of the cow (Patterson *et al.,* 2003). Feeds should contain at least 0.1 ppm selenium on a dry matter basis (Pradhan and Nakaghosi, 2003). In some herds, feed sources must be supplemented with selenium injections to maintain blood levels above the recommended 8-10 mg/100 ml. After injection, feed supplements may provide enough selenium to maintain adequate blood levels in the cow. Blood tests are recommended to confirm selenium status when questions arise.

Zinc (Zn)

The essential component of over 200 enzyme systems is zinc in which the metabolic action includes carbohydrate and protein metabolism, protein synthesis, nucleic acid metabolism, epithelial tissue integrity, cell repair, cell division, vitamin A and E transport and utilization (Wichtell *et al.*, 1996). In addition, zinc also plays a major role in the immune system and certain reproductive hormones (Capuco *et al.*, 1990). Zinc is known to be essential for proper sexual maturity, reproductive capacity, and more specifically, onset of oestrus. Zinc has a critical role in the repair and maintenance of the uterine lining following parturition, speeding return to normal reproductive function and oestrus (Goff, 1999). Zinc deficiency results in poor semen quality and reduced testicular size and libido in bulls (Daniel, 1983). It has also increases plasma beta carotene levels. Increased plasma beta carotene has been directly correlated to improved conception rates and embryonic development (Staats *et al.*, 1988). Insufficient zinc supplementation results in mild to severe claw (hoof) disorders, including weak claws that are more susceptible to inter-digital and digital dermatitis and foot rot (Patterson *et al.*,2003). The recommended dietary content of zinc for dairy cattle is typically between 18 and 73ppm depending upon the stage of development and dry matter intake (NRC, 2001). Zinc supplementation also raises the ejaculate volume, sperm concentration, percent live sperm and percent sperm motility in crossbred bulls (Dunn and Moss, 1992).

Copper (Cu)

Copper is a vital trace element for normal hemoglobin synthesis in young rabbits and rats. The importance of Cu for normal growth, production and reproductive performance has also been established. The biological role of Cu is exerted through a number of Cu-containing proteins including ceruloplasmin and superoxide dismutase (SOD) (Prohaska and Lukasewycz, 1990). Copper is also necessary component of various enzymes including superoxide dismutase, lysyl oxidase and thiol oxidase. These enzymes function to eliminate free radicals that increase tissue susceptibility to bacterial infections, increase structural strength and elasticity of connective tissues and blood vessels and increase strength of horn such as in the claw (Hoof), minimizing lameness (Nix *et al.*, 1981). Symptoms of a copper deficiency include early embryonic death, resorption of embryo, increased retained placentas and necrosis of the placenta (Patterson *et al.,* 2003). Dairy cows with higher serum copper levels had significantly less days to first service, fewer services per conception and fewer days to open (Jousan *et al.,* 2002). In male proper copper supplementation is needed for production of quality semen (Patterson *et al.,* 2003). When Cu is inadequate in animals, physiological and metabolic functions related to the Cu-enzymes may be impaired and, during clinical deficiency, symptoms will appear. Although low Cu content of feedstuffs is a common cause of Cu inadequacy, reducing bioavailability of Cu in ruminants may occur when dietary sulphur, molybdenum, zinc or iron are high (Hemken *et al.,* 1998).

Manganese (Mn)

Manganese is an activator of enzyme systems in the metabolism of carbohydrate, fats, protein and nucleic acids (Patterson *et al.,* 2003). Manganese appears to have a vital role in reproduction. It is necessary for cholesterol synthesis (Kappel and Zidenberg, 1999), which in turn is required for synthesis of the steroids, estrogen, progesterone and testosterone. Insufficient steroid production results in decreased circulating concentrations of these reproductive hormones resulting in abnormal sperm in males and irregular estrus cycles in females. The corpus luteum has high manganese content and may be affected by level of manganese supplementation. Also, vaginal manganese concentration is higher in cycling than in anoestrous ruminants. A deficiency in manganese may be associated with suppression of estrus, cystic ovaries and reduced conception rate (Patterson *et al.,* 2003).

Cobalt (Co)

Cobalt is needed for vitamin B12 synthesis. Maintaining adequate vitamin B12 status benefits both the dam and offspring. When adequate, sufficient amounts of vitamin B12 cross the placenta and are present in colostrums (Nix *et al.,* 1981). Milk and colostrums in particular, contain high levels of vitamin B12 which is required for the conversion of propionate to glucose and for folic acid metabolism. Diminution of cobalt and vitamin B12 during parturition causes depressed milk production and colostrums yield and quality (Patterson *et al.,* 2003). Cobalt deficiency reduces fertility and sub-optimal conditionings of the offspring are noted. Inadequate cobalt levels in the diet have been correlated with increased early calf mortality. A cobalt deficiency ultimately results in a vitamin B_{12} deficiency. Manganese, zinc, iodine and monensin may reduce cobalt deficiency (Patterson *et al.,* 2003).

Iodine (I)

Iodine is required for synthesis of thyroid hormone, thyroxin, which regulates the rate of metabolism (NRC, 2001). The iodine is also essential for initiation of follicular wave dynamic, ovarian activities, release of best quality mature oocytes and improvement of rate of service per conception in dairy cows (Sarkar, 2006). Reproduction is influenced through iodine's action on the thyroid gland. Inadequate thyroid function reduces conception rate and ovarian activity. Thus, iodine deficiency impairs reproduction and iodine supplementation has been suggested when necessary to insure that cows consume 15-20 mg of iodine each day. Excessive iodine intakes have been associated with various health problems including abortion and decreased resistance to infection and disease. Signs of subclinical iodine deficiency in breeding females include suppressed oestrus, abortions, still births, increased frequency of retained placenta and extended gestation periods (Hess *et al.,*2008). Calves born to cows that are marginally deficient in iodine are weak and may be hairless (Patterson *et al.,* 2003). Besides, animals that have a subclinical iodine deficiency will also have increased incidence of foot rot and respiratory disease due to suppressed immune responses. One distinguished characteristic of a clinical iodine deficiency is an enlargement of the thyroid gland, often termed as gaiter (Hess *et al.,* 2008).

Iron (Fe)

Iron is required for the synthesis of haemoglobin and myoglobin as well as many enzymes and cytochrome enzymes of electron transport chain (Kumar *et al.,* 2011). Iron functions in transport of oxygen to tissues, maintenance of oxidative enzyme system and is concerned with ferreting formation (Khilare *et al.,* 2007). Deficiency in adult animals is rare due to its pervasive presence in the feed stuffs. The reproductive performance of iron deficient animals may be badly affected due to anaemia, reduced appetite and lower body condition. A deficient animal becomes repeat breeders and required increased number of inseminations per conception and occasionally may abort.

Potassium (K)

Recent research suggests that feeding high levels of potassium may delay the onset of puberty, delay ovulation, impair corpus luteum (yellow body) development and increase the incidence of anoestrus in heifers. Schweigert and Zucker (1988) reported that lower fertility in cows fed with high levels of potassium or diets in which the potassium-sodium ratio was too wide.

Chromium (Cr)

Chromium potentiates insulin action, resulting in increased uptake of glucose and amino acids by cells in the body (Short and Adams, 1988). A chromium deficiency in lactating cows may result in increased incidence of ketosis and decreased milk production. Improved energy balance in early lactation may improve reproduction (Patterson *et al.,* 2003). Chromium also plays an important role in the secretion of pregnancy specific proteins from the uterine endometrium which is helpful in preventing early embryonic death. Chromium exerts a significant influence on follicular maturation and LH release. It can possibly lead to lower sperm count and decreased fertility and influences foetal growth and development. (Tuormaa, 2000).

Molybdenum (Mo)

Molybdenum is co-dependent with Cu with reference to body system of ruminants. Generally lower level of one occurs in presence toxic level of another. Therefore proper balance of Cu and Mo in soil and plants is essential for normal absorption of each other in ruminants (Randhawa and Randhawa, 1994). Molybdenum deficiency decreases libido, reduced spermatogenesis and causes sterility in males and is responsible for delayed puberty, reduced conception rate and anoestrus in females (Kumar *et al.,* 2011).

Salt (Sodium and Chloride)

Salt deficiencies can affect the efficiency of digestion and indirectly the reproduction performance of cows (Short and Adams, 1988). Sodium and chloride normally do not appear in feedstuffs in adequate amounts to meet animal requirements and should be provided free choice at all times (Elrod and Butler, 1993).

Summary

It is clear that the macro and micro minerals have a great impact on animal's reproductive physiology and its imbalance causes various problems leading to lowered reproductive efficiency as well as repeat breeding. Adequate minerals supplementation is required as most of the roughages, greens, concentrate and even most of commercial feeds are deficient in trace mineral elements. The best recommendation at present is to provide a feeding program for productive animals which is balanced for all minerals and meets all known requirements and of course it should be area specific.

Table 1. Normal value of certain blood biochemical constituents in cattle (Jackson and Cockcroft, 2002)

Serum constituents	Normal range
Calcium, total (mg/dL)	9.7-12.4
Calcium, ionised (mg/dL)	4.8- 6.2
Phosphorus (mg/dL)	5.6-8.0
Magnesium (mg/dL)	1.8-2.3
Iron (mg/dL)	57-162
Potassium (mmol/L)	3.9-5.8
Sodium (mmol/L)	132-152
Chloride (mmol/L)	95-110

Chapter-4

Role of Nutrients for the Management of Repeat Breeding

Livestock production efficiency or productivity is to a large extent dependent on reproductive performance. Several factors are known to affect the reproductive performance of farm animals, among which are biological type, the physical environment and nutrition. Nutrition is recognized as a modulator of reproductive function. Energy and protein are the major nutrients required in the greatest amounts and should be in the topmost priority in order to optimize reproduction in dairy cattle. In the other hand, Level of feeding and bodyweight also affects fertility. The report by various researchers suggested that malnutrition resulting from inadequate, excess or imbalanced nutrients intake may delay puberty, reduce ovulation, lower conception rates, compromise embryonic and fetal survival, result in poor lactation, lengthen post partum anestrus and reduce perinatal survival as well as performance which may lead to repeat breeding (Bazer *et al.,* 2014). In case of tropical countries most of the animals are fed with high roughage based diet. To achieve noble performance improving their feeding with adequate nutrient supply can immediately increase their reproductive performance.

Relationships of Dietary Protein and Fertility

Protein is the main constituent of building block element. Excess or deficiency of this constituent leads to detrimental effect to the body. As a nutrient, protein provides amino acids for the animal to build its own proteins. Of the 20 amino acids used to make proteins, only 10 of these can be synthesized in sufficient quantity to meet the animal's demands for amino acids. The other 10, which are termed essential amino acids, must be obtained from the diet. In dairy cattle and other ruminants, there are two main sources of amino acids. Much of the protein in the diet is degraded in the rumen called as rumen degradable protein (RDP) and is used by the microbes in the rumen for synthesis of their own proteins. When the microbes pass to the small intestine, microbial proteins are broken down and are used by the cow. This fraction of dietary protein is called microbial protein. The dietary protein not used by rumen microbes is available for digestion in the small intestine and is called rumen undegradable protein (RUP). The percent of dietary protein that is not degraded in the rumen can vary greatly depending on the feedstuff and ranges from 0-80%.The microbial protein (truly digestible amino acids in microbes from the rumen) and rumen undegraded protein (RUP *i.e.*, the truly digestible amino acids in feed protein that has bypassed the rumen) are the sources of metabolisable protein (MP), which is essentially the amino acids absorbed from the small intestine. It is essential that the animals should be given adequate protein during the post weaning period to get optimum growth and early puberty. It is also well recognized that an increase in prepubertal LH pulse frequency is an important event for the onset of puberty (Kaur and Arora, 1995). Attention is now being paid to the cellular biochemical changes being mediated through certain amino acids which influence pulsatile LH secretion. Thus it is necessary to make this distinction as the balance (dietary supply relative to requirement) of these different protein fractions may have different effects on fertility. Sufficient circulating concentrations of amino acids, particularly rate-limiting amino acids such as methionine and lysine are critical for optimal milk production. Generally the first three rate-limiting amino acids for milk production are considered to be Methionine, Lysine, and Histidine. In addition, many amino acids can have positive effects on physiological processes that are independent of their effects on synthesis of proteins. This has been termed "functional effects" of amino acids and methionine and arginine effects are the best studied "functional amino acids" that have been linked to reproduction (Penagaricano *et al.*, 2013, Hansen, 2016). The rate-limiting amino acids may also impact embryonic development, perhaps through improved amino acid profiles in the uterine lumen. Methionine may also have direct epigenetic effects in the embryo by methylation of DNA (Wiltbank *et al.*, 2014).

Various published research, indicated that feeding excess RDP has a negative effect on fertility (Gunn et al., 2016). Tamminga (2006) clearly states that feeding high levels of RDP delays the first ovulation or oestrus, reduces the conception rate to first insemination, increases the number of days open and lowers the overall conception rate. There are several proposed mechanisms for this effect including an exacerbated NEB (Negative Energy Balance) for cows fed diets high in RDP in comparison to diets high in RUP (Gunn *et al.*, 2014b) and proven deleterious effects of both ammonia and urea on both oocyte and embryo development (Ocon and Hansen, 2003; Rhoads *et al.*, 2006). Dietary excesses of MP are thought to be of lesser consequence than excesses of RDP in terms of dairy cow fertility, excess MP supply relative to requirement will often increase milk yield and exacerbate NEB. Hence supply relatively low amounts of MP, in order to reduce milk yield response to energy supplementation and thus improve energy balance.

Feeding high protein diets increases urea and ammonia levels in the blood along with ovarian follicles and the uterus. Urea circulating in the blood stream is measured as urea nitrogen in either plasma (PUN) or serum fractions and is often referred to generically as blood urea nitrogen (BUN). Measurements of PUN or MUN have provided a useful index for studying the association between metabolism of dietary protein and reproductive efficiency. This high urea nitrogen, measured in blood or milk is associated with reduced fertility in dairy cows along with costs, environmental impacts, and efficiency of nitrogen utilization (Sinclair *et al.*, 2014). High urea concentrations exert direct effects on the uterine luminal environment.

Overfeeding protein during the breeding season and early gestation, particularly if the rumen receives an inadequate supply of energy may be associated with decreased fertility. This decrease in fertility may result from decreased uterine pH during the luteal phase of the estrous cycle in cattle fed high levels of degradable protein. The combined effect of elevated urea and negative energy balance impairs the viability of embryos in lactating cows and contributes to lower fertility (Butler, 1998). Pregnancy rates were decreased by about 20% when PUN (Plasma Urea Nitrogrn) or MUN (Milk Urea Nitrogen) was >19 mg/dl (Butler, 2005).

Feeding protein and urea, such that early lactating cows have a diet containing 16% protein and late lactating cows have a diet containing 12% protein, should optimize the fertility of the cows. Urea also advances blastocyst hatching (Wiltbank *et al.*, 2014) that could result in asynchrony between the embryo and uterine environment. In addition elevated ammonia in the uterine lumen of cows fed high dietary protein may directly impair embryo development (Hammon *et al.*, 2004). Also elevated urea level of in the blood consequently leads to alteration of hormonal balances mainly lower progesterone levels in the blood or by interfering with the normal inductive effects of progesterone on the uterine micro environment, thereby providing suboptimal conditions for the support of embryo development (Butler, 2005, Wiltbank *et al.*, 2014).

Table 2. Effect of protein on progesterone concentration (Yasothai, 2014)

Control	Progesterone level (ng/ml)
Control	3.8
13% protein	6.5
22% protein	2.5

Energy

Among the various nutrients energy balance is one of the most important nutritional factors related to poor reproductive function in farm animals. In both breeding and nonbreeding females nutrient acquisition must satisfy conflicting requirements for maintenance, growth, and reproduction that demand different types of tissue production over different time period along with nutrient partitioning for milk production. Based on this list of metabolic priorities for energy, reproductive function is compromised because available energy is directed towards meeting minimum energy reserves and milk production. High producing dairy cows need to mobilize body reserve to be able to sustain their milk production. In early lactation, until energy intake assures the requirements, dairy cows, especially high producing breeds, enter a state of negative energy balance (NEB), losing high amounts of body condition. Due to the deficiency of dietary energy of high yielding animals during first lactation leads to mobilization of body reserves for production purpose affects reproductive status by increasing the length of the time interval to first ovulation (Nishany *et al.*, 2013). Pirestani and Maybodi (2015) reported that adequate energy diet has beneficial effect on steroid hormone (estrogen and progesterone), and reproduction indices in

Holstein heifers. Research has shown that cows will ovulate approximately 10 days after reaching the lowest point of negative energy balance (Robinson *et al.,* 2006). Metabolic status impacts reproductive function at systemic level, modulating the hypothalamic GnRH neuronal network and/or the pituitary gonadotropin secretion through several hormones and neuropeptides, and at the ovarian level, acting through the regulation of follicle growth and steroidogenesis by means of the growth hormone-IGF-insulin system and local ovarian mediators. Potential sites of action of nutrition on ovarian function include systemic effects at the hypothalamic level via GnRH synthesis and release; the anterior pituitary through control of synthesis and release of FSH, LH, and growth hormone (GH); at the ovarian level through regulation of follicle growth and steroid synthesis. Growth of follicles and ovulation are dependent on the pulsatile secretion of LH (Garcia, 2012). In cattle in severe negative energy balance inhibited the secretion of LH hormone (Wathes *et al.,* 2007). Disrupted or decreased LH secretion slows the growth and development of the follicle, which delays ovulation. Metabolic hormones such as leptin, insulin and insulin like growth factor-I (IGF-I) are also required for normal follicular growth and ovulation. They either suppress or stimulate developing follicles in a concentration-dependent manner (Do and Taylor, 2015). Cows in negative energy balance have reduced levels of IGF-I. This is an important relationship, given that IGF-I amplify the effects of LH on the ovary through potentiating the signalling mechanism for LH ((Diskin *et al.,* 2003). Therefore, the actions of LH are decreased in cows in negative energy balance because lower IGF-I leads to reduced effectiveness of LH. Consequently, follicles in cows with extremely low IGF-I do not develop normally, and ovulation is delayed because LH is less active. This effect was demonstrated in a study by Kirsz and Zieba (2012).

The other possible effects of deficient energy intake are lower conception rates, longer calving intervals, underdeveloped mammary glands, greater incidence of calving problems and cystic ovaries which are most prevalent in high producing dairy cows that are in negative energy balance common link between this disease and negative energy balance is the abnormal secretion of LH (Chagas *et al.,* 2007). Cystic ovaries are associated with increased LH secretion but an inhibition of the preovulatory LH surge. The cumulative effect of these conditions is development of a large cystic follicle that fails to ovulate in the absence of the ovulatory surge of LH. This relationship further strengthens the relationship among energy balance, LH and early postpartum reproductive performance of the dairy cow. Restricting energy intake during late gestation increases the length of postpartum anestrous and reduces subsequent pregnancy rate. The impact of insufficient energy intake during late gestation cannot be overcome by increasing energy intake postpartum (Butler, 2014). Inadequate energy intake in heifers will lead to delay in sexual maturity (Youngquist and Threlfall, 2007). Also excess energy intake may also harmful during late lactation and the dry period. It can cause "fat cow" problems which lower reproductive efficiency in the next lactation. But the impact of a short-term increase in energy intake (flushing) on the numbers of cows cycling or pregnancy rate may be dependent on the previous nutritional status of the cow. Reduction of energy demands by short-term (48 hour) after calving combined with flushing can reduce days to oestrus and improve conception rates (Robinson *et al.*, 2006). Caution should be used with feeding excessive amounts of nutrients before or after calving. Not only it is costly, but animals with excess body condition score (BCS >7) have lower reproductive performance and more calving difficulty than animals in moderate body condition (BCS 5-6) (Chandra *et al.*, 2011). Overfeeding often results in weak expression of estrus, subnormal conception rates, high embryonic mortality, decreased mammary gland development and reduced milk production (Berry *et al.*, 2016). Cows that are over-conditioned when they calve have a higher incidence of retained placenta, more uterine infections and more cystic ovaries. They also have a higher incidence of metabolic disorders and have a greater tendency to go off feed. All of these problems can result in poor reproductive performance.

Effects of dietary fatty acids on reproduction in ruminants

Addition fats and fatty acids in the diet have some specific effect on the endocrine function of the animal which may act directly on the reproductive axis. Supplementing fat to improve reproduction was initially attempted to increase the energy density in the diet. Fats are highly digestible (approximately 80% digestible). In general, the amount of added fat in predominantly forage-based cattle diets should not exceed 6% of the total ration on a dry matter basis. However, high levels of fat in the diet have the potential to negatively impact fibre digestibility, decrease calcium absorption by formation of calcium salts of fatty acids, and increase vitamin E requirements (NRC, 2001).

If a higher energy level is needed, then bypass fat could be added to fulfil the needed energy requirement. Provide adequate calcium in the ration, and make sure the vitamin E content meets or exceeds requirements, especially when highly unsaturated oils are used. Most of the fats fed to cattle are in the form of triacyl glycerols in plant and animal products or as free FA or FA saponified to Ca in processed fat supplements. Several fatty acid sources have been studied as they relate to reproductive function. Common sources include sunflower, safflower, cottonseed, rice bran, soybeans, fishmeal, animal tallow, and calcium salts of fatty acids. Fats of plant or animal origin contain the unsaturated fatty acids palmitoleic, oleic, linoleic, and á-linolenic acids. Rodney *et al.* (2015) from meta-analysis of transition animal data reported the effects specific fatty acids in dietary interventions that contribute to increasing fertility of cows but did not identify the reasons for these improvements in regard to the FA composition of the diet. Linoleic acid is found mainly in oilseeds, whereas linolenic acid is found predominantly in forages and in some oilseeds (e.g. flaxseed); Eicosapentaenoic and docosahexaenoic acids are high in fish oils. Dairy cows fed diets high in eicosapentaenoic and docosahexaenoic acids (supplementation with menhaden fish meal) or linolenic acid (supplementation with flaxseed) during early pregnancy had reduced PGF2 production and increased pregnancy rates. Feeding diets high in linolenic acid during the dry period may increase the incidence of placental retention.

Fats in the diet can influence reproduction positively by altering both ovarian follicle and corpus luteum function via improved energy status and by increasing precursors for the synthesis of reproductive hormones such as steroids and prostaglandins. Dietary fats favor reproductive function by supplying energy and by actions on reproductive processes that are not related to energy. For example, increased availability of fatty acid precursors allows increased steroid and eicosanoid secretion, which can alter ovarian and uterine function and affect pregnancy rates. At the cell, fatty acids may have a direct effect on the transcription of genes that encode proteins that are essential to reproductive events.

Mechanisms through which fat supplementation could enhance reproduction in farm animal

Fats are hydrolyzed in the rumen to their polyunsaturated fatty acid constituents and glycerol. The consumption of polyunsaturated plant oils increases basal serum insulin concentrations in cattle. It is possible that increased serum concentrations of insulin may play a role in mediating increased follicular growth either directly or indirectly by modulating granulosa IGF-I (insulin-like growth factor–1) production. Fat supplementation has also been shown to increase concentration of circulating growth hormone (Ryan *et al.*, 2014). Secretion of luteinizing hormone (LH) from the pituitary and follicular growth in cattle are regulated partially by the energy status of the animal. Energy provided by fat supplementation increases LH secretion in animals deficient in energy. A mechanism independent from energy by which dietary fatty acids affect LH secretion has not been established (Mattos *et al.*, 2000). Feeding supplemental dietary fat also increased serum and follicular fluid cholesterol, serum progesterone, lifespan of induced corpus luteum (CL), the number of medium-sized follicles, and growth of the preovulatory follicle. Prostaglandins play an important role in reestablishing estrous cycles both immediately after parturition and thereafter until conception occurs. Prostaglandin F2α (PGF2α) is responsible for uterine involution after parturition. The greater postpartum prostaglandin concentration, faster the uterine involution. The uterus releases PGF2α during each estrous to regress each new CL if the cow is not pregnant and initiate a new estrous cycle. During the period of CL regression, concentrations of PGF2α and progesterone are inversely related. If the cow does conceive, release of PGF2α from the uterus is prevented in order to preserve the CL and maintain pregnancy. The fatty acid, linoleic acid is a substrate for the synthesis of PGF2α. Linoleic acid can inhibit prostaglandin synthesis by competitive inhibition with these key enzymes. Arachidonic, and two fatty acids found in fishmeal, eicosapentaenoic (C20:5) and docosahexanoic (C22:6), have been shown to inhibit cyclooxygenase activity as well. It is important to note that linolenic acid (C18:3) was also present in the endometrial prostaglandin synthesis inhibitor isolated by Thatcher *et al.* (2011), and that linolenic acid has been shown to be a strong inhibitor of prostaglandin synthesis. The amount and probably type of particular fatty acids reaching the target tissues likely influence whether prostaglandin synthesis is stimulated or inhibited (Thatcher and Staples, 2000). Also manipulation of the fatty acid profile of the diet can be used potentially to amplify suppression of uterine synthesis of prostaglandin F2á during early pregnancy in cattle, which may contribute to a reduction in embryonic mortality (Rahbar *et al.*, 2014).

Summary

It is clear that nutrition is directly related to reproduction in the dairy cow. Nutrient either in deficient amount or in higher amount has been shown to be capable of altering reproduction which leads to infertility and ultimately repeat breeding. The basic problem is that the degree of the excess, deficiency or imbalance which is required to alter reproduction is still unclear. The best recommendation at present is to provide a feeding program for dairy cows which is balanced for all nutrients and meets all known nutrient requirements. Dietary improvements to pasture and forage plants should be considered since they are a very cost-effective way to enhance animal reproductive performance as well as it minimises the incidence of repeat breeding.

❑❑❑

Chapter-5

Genital Changes in Different Categories of Repeat Breeder Cow

The genital tract of non-pregnant cows normally lies in the pelvic cavity and consists of the vulva, vagina, cervix, uterus, Fallopian tubes (oviducts), ovaries and their supporting structures (Figure 4). The reproductive structures can be palpated through the rectum and this is the basis of routine fertility work. In general the reproductive tract of *Bos indicus* cattle is smaller than that of taurine cattle. Before going to rectal palpation one should know the normal location and structure of the genital tract of the cow. In this regard, the normal shape and size of the genital tract of the cow is discussed.

The uterus is a muscular type of organ which consisting of a body, about 4 to 5 cm long, and two uterine horns (cornua), each 15 to 25 cm in length and 1 to 3 cm in diameter. The uterus is suspended by the broad ligament in a coiled or curled manner. Its size varies with breed, age, parity, pregnancy and disease.

The cervix is a sphincter-like structure with a thick wall and a narrow lumen. This lumen is tightly closed, except during oestrus and at parturition, and the cervix forms a barrier between the uterus and the outside environment. The length of the cervix varies from 1.5 cm in heifers to 8 cm in multiparous cows of larger breeds. Interlocking ridges and complex folding of the lumen mucosa can hamper insertion of a pipette or tube for intra-uterine insemination or infusions.

The vagina extends backwards from the cervix and opens into the vulva. Its length varies with breed and stage of pregnancy. The vaginal epithelial cells near the cervix secrete mucus, especially around the time of oestrus.

The ovaries are oval-shaped structures, 1 to 4 cm long and 1 to 3 cm in diameter; their size depends on the stage of the reproductive cycle. They are linked to the uterus by the Fallopian tubes which open anteriorly into the fimbriae - funnel-shaped structures close to, but not attached to the ovaries. The fimbriae guide unfertilized eggs from the ovary into the Fallopian tubes.

Regarding oestrus signs, the most common physical signs of oestrus are hyperemia and oedema of vulva and mucus discharge from the vulva (Morrow, 1969). There is presence of a mature follicle and increased uterine tone. According to Zemjanis (1970) a fully developed corpus luteum and absence of follicle of significant size in the ovary indicated 8th to 16th day of the oestrous cycle in cattle. The vulva became relaxed and oedematous during oestrus, vaginal mucosa became pink and congested and strings of mucus hung from the vulva (Roberts, 1971). The Graafian follicle becomes larger and matured during oestrus. The corpus luteum attained maximum size of 2 to 2.5 cm by 7 to 8 days after ovulation. Sukh Deo and Roy (1971) reported that the colour of mucus in normal as well as repeat breeding cows remained clean. Consistency of mucus appeared thin and thick in 50.4 and 49.6 per cent cases respectively in normal cows and 52.3 and 47.7 per cent respectively in repeaters. The absence of corpus luteum from day 9 to 12 of the oestrous cycle in repeat breeding cows was indicative of anovulatory oestrus as stated by Kavani and Kodagali (1984). The cervical mucus secretion during oestrus was stimulated by ovarian oestrogen and inhibited by progesterone (Hafez, 1987). The follicular growth, ovulation and luteal functions are regulated by the hypothalamo- pituitary-ovarian axis and the physicochemical properties of cervical mucus were altered under the influence of oestrogen. Oestrogen was also reported to cause dilatation of the cervix and increased tonacity of the uterus (Jainudeen and Hafez, 1987). Deshpande (1994) stated that the uterine tonacity in cattle increased due to tropic action of oestrogen. Oestrogen also caused gradual relaxation of the cervix during oestrus. Das (2002) observed that the cows with anovulatory oestrus; the swelling of vulva and pink colourations of the vaginal mucous membrane (Figure 5, 6) occurred in 5% and 25% respectively and these were observed upto 48 hours of oestrus. He also stated that animals with anovulation had clear vaginal mucus discharge during the oestrus period and the uterus remained tonus upto 48 hours of oestrus. There may be palpable of Graafian follicle till 48 hours of oestrus. The consistency and patency of the cervix as relaxed and open in all (100%) repeat breeding cattle with anovulation and delayed ovulation upto 24 hours of oestrus as reported by Das (2005). Talukdar *et al.* (2013) in their study stated that the congestion of vulvar mucous membrane persisted upto day 1 of oestrus in all repeat breeder cows with anovulation, delayed ovulation and normal ovulation (Table 3-5). The vaginal discharge on day 0 was found free flowing in higher percentage of cows with anoulation (70.00%) and normal ovulation (83.33%). The 50 per cent cows with delayed ovulation showed free flowing vaginal discharge on the day of oestrus. Up to day 2 of oestrus the cervix remained open in all cows (100%) with anovulation and delayed ovulation while it was closed in all cows with normal ovulation by that time. Uterine tone was good in 63.33 per cent cows with anovulation and normal ovulation as against 40.00 per cent cows with delayed ovulation on day 1 of oestrus. They also indicated that common signs of oestrus such as congestion of vulvar mucous membrane, free flowing vaginal discharge (Figure 7), good uterine tone and patency of the cervix were prolonged in cows affected with anovulation and delayed ovulation.

Summary

It is obvious that Vulva remained congested upto day 1 of oestrus in the repeat breeder cow with anovulation, delayed ovulation and normal ovulation. Free flowing vaginal discharge was also seen on day 0 of oestrus in anovulatory cows. The cervix remained open upto day 2 of oestrus in repeat breeder cows with anovlation and delayed ovulation and upto day 1 of oestrus in normal ovulation. Good uterine tone was detected upto day 1 of oestrus in repeat breeder cows with anovlation and normal ovulation. The animals with anovulation had clear vaginal mucus discharge during the oestrus period and the uterus remained tonus upto 48 hours of oestrus. There may be palpable of Graafian follicle till 48 hours of oestrus. The corpus luteum was palpable on day 8 of oestrus in cows with delayed and normal ovulation but not in anovulation. The absence of corpus luteum from day 9 to 12 of the oestrous cycle in repeat breeding cows was indicative of anovulatory oestrus.

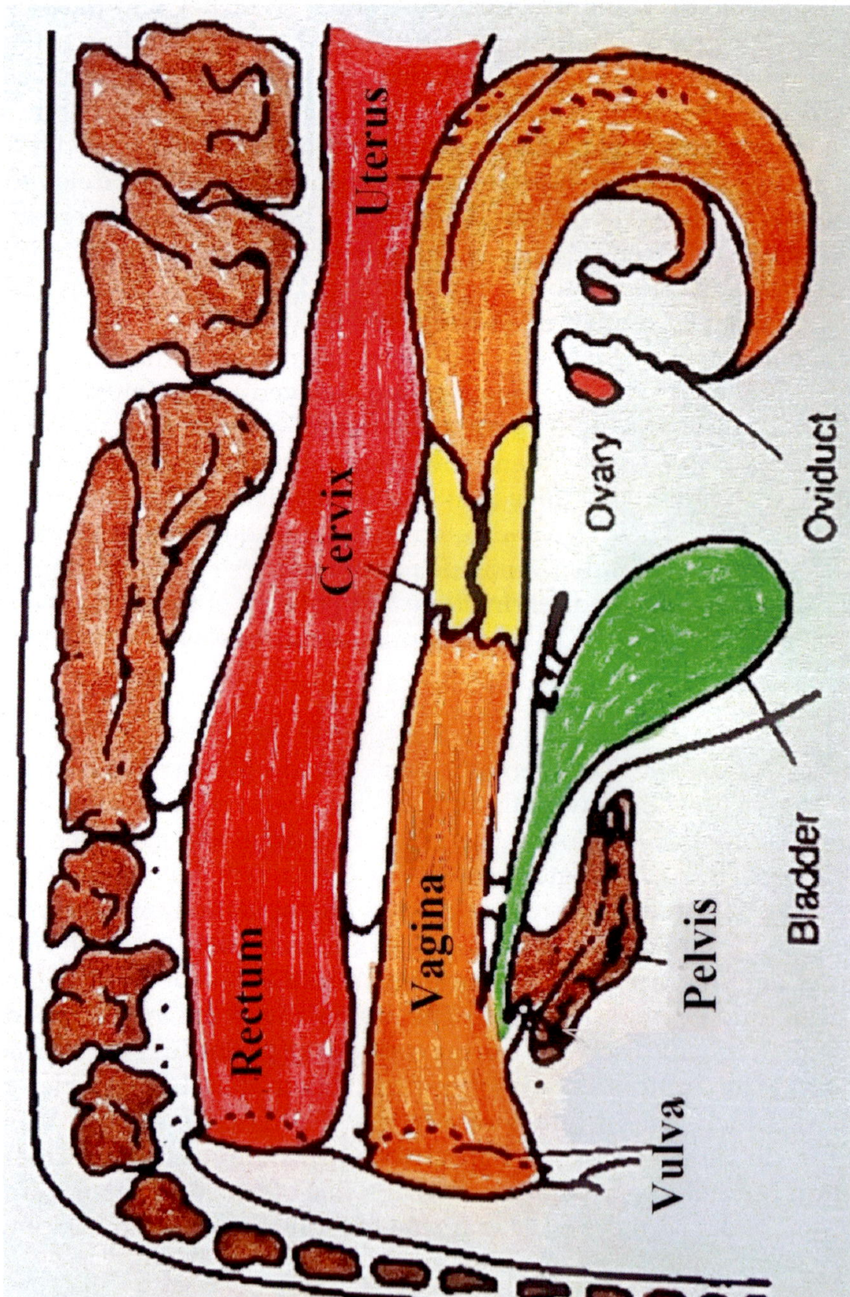

Figure 4. Normal position of cow genital organ

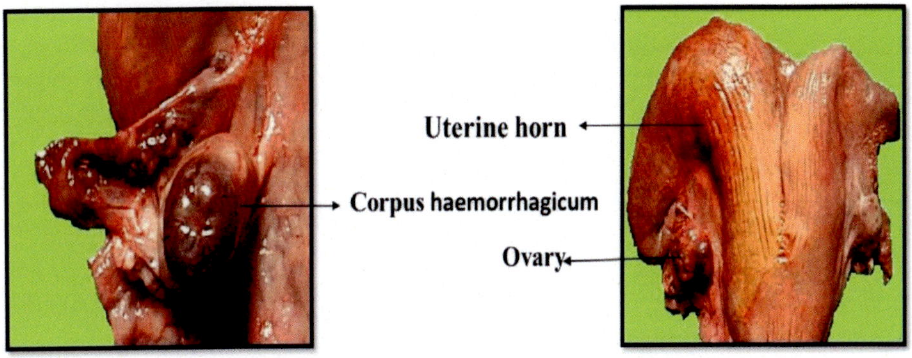

Figure 5. Genital organ of a cow

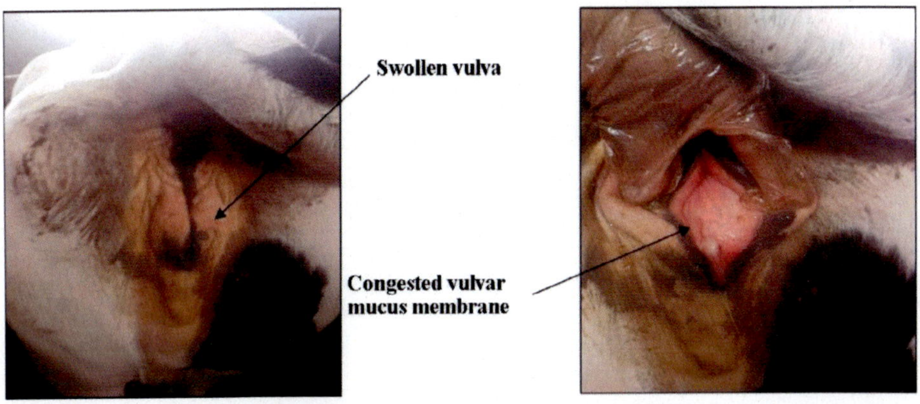

Figure 6. Oestrus signs of a cow

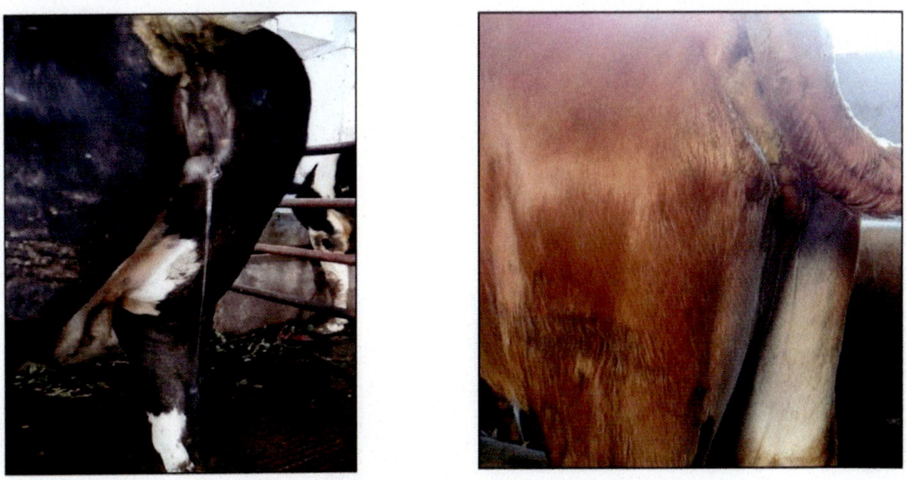

Figure 7. Transparent and abundant vaginal mucus indicates optimal heat and good uterine environment

Table 3. Genital changes at day 0, 1, 2 and 8 of oestrus in repeat breeder crossbred cows with anovulation (n=30) (Talukdar *et al.*, 2013)

Reproductive organ	Condition	Frequency of occurrence (%)			
		Day 0	Day 1	Day 2	Day 8
Vulva	Congestion of vulva	100.00(30)	96.66(29)	3.33(1)	—
	Absent	—	3.33(1)	96.66(29)	100.00(30)
Vagina	Free flowing vaginal discharge	70.00(21)	40.00(12)	6.66(2)	—
	Medium vaginal discharge	16.66(5)	10.00(3)	—	—
	Absent	13.33(4)	50.00(15)	93.33(28)	100.00(30)
Cervix	Open	96.66(29)	100.00(30)	100.00(30)	—
	Closed	3.33(1)	—	—	100.00(30)
Uterus	Good tone	63.33(19)	63.33(19)	13.33(4)	—
	Moderate tone	33.33(10)	33.33(10)	80.00(24)	16.66(5)
	No tone	3.33(1)	3.33(1)	6.66(2)	83.33(25)
Ovary	Graafian follicle	100.00(30)	100.00(30)	100.00(30)	—
	Corpus haemorrhagicum	—	—	—	—
	Mature corpus luteum	—	—	—	—

Figures in the parentheses indicate number of animals.

Table 4. Genital changes at day 0, 1, 2 and 8 of oestrus in repeat breeder crossbred cows with delayed ovulation (n=20) (Talukdar *et al.*, 2013)

Reproductive organ	Condition	Frequency of occurrence (%)			
		Day 0	Day 1	Day 2	Day 8
Vulva	Congestion of vulva	100.00(20)	90.00(18)	5.00(1)	__
	Absent	___	10.00(2)	95.00(19)	100.00(20)
Vagina	Free flowing vaginal discharge	50.00(10)	40.00(8)	5.00(1)	___
	Medium vaginal discharge	25.00(5)	40.00(8)	5.00(1)	___
	Absent	25.00(5)	20.00(4)	90.00(18)	100.00(20)
Cervix	Open	90.00(18)	100.00(20)	100.00(20)	___
	Closed	10.00(2)	___	___	100.00(20)
Uterus	Good tone	40.00(8)	40.00(8)	____	___
	Moderate tone	50.00(10)	60.00(12)	80.00(16)	20.00(4)
	No tone	10.00(2)	___	20.00(4)	80.00(16)
Ovary	Graafian follicle	100.00(20)	100.00(20)	100.00(20)	___
	Corpus haemorrhagicum	___	____	10.00(2)	__
	Mature corpus luteum	___	___	___	100.00(20)

Figures in the parentheses indicate number of animals.

Table 5. Genital changes at day 0, 1, 2 and 8 of oestrus in repeat breeder crossbred cows with normal ovulation (n=30) (Talukdar *et al.*, 2013)

Reproductive organ	Condition	Frequency of occurrence (%)			
		Day 0	Day 1	Day 2	Day 8
Vulva	Congestion of vulva	100.00(30)	96.66(29)	___	__
	Absent	___	3.33(1)	100.00(30)	100.00(30)
Vagina	Free flowing vaginal discharge	83.33(25)	40.00(12)	___	___
	Medium vaginal discharge	10.00(3)	10.00(3)	6.66(2)	___
	Absent	6.66(2)	50.00(15)	93.33(28)	100.00(30)
Cervix	Open	96.66(29)	100.00(30)	___	___
	Closed	3.33(1)	___	100.00(30)	100.00(30)
Uterus	Good tone	66.66(20)	63.33(19)	___	___
	Moderate tone	33.33(10)	36.66(11)	80.00(24)	6.66(2)
	No tone	___	___	20.00(6)	93.33(28)
Ovary	Graafian follicle	100.00(30)	___	___	___
	Corpus haemorrhagicum	___	100.00(30)	___	___
	Mature corpus luteum	___	___	___	100.00(30)

Figures in the parentheses indicate number of animals.

❑❑❑

Chapter-6

Blood Biochemical Profile of Repeat Breeder Dairy Cattle

Repeat breeding is one of the major problems in dairy cattle that affects fertility and in turn incurs great economic loss to farmers. It has multi-factorial etiology such as infectious or inflammatory processes, nutritional deficiencies, managemental practices, ovulatory disturbances *etc.* (Gunther, 1981). Mineral imbalance or deficiencies is another important cause of repeat breeding in cattle (Rupde *et al.*, 1993; Das *et al.*, 2002). Variations in the level of trace elements have been found to be associated with reproductive disorders (Jain and Madan, 1984; Jain, 1993) and similar findings was also reported by the author (Table 6). The deficiency of a particular element may influence the level of other elements in the body fluid and the functional characteristics of endocrine glands, especially the hypophyseal-gonadal axis (Bhaskaran and Abdullakhan, 1981).

Calcium (Ca) plays an important role to sensitizing the tubular genitalia for the action of hormone there by increasing the fertility rate in the animals (Moddie, 1965). Calcium is also responsible for steroidogenesis by influencing delivery or utilization of cholesterol by mitochondria or by stimulating the conversion of pregnenolone to progesterone (Seifi *et al.*, 2005). In repeat breeder cows the average calcium values ranged from 10.04 ± 0.32 mg to 8.24 ± 0.22 mg per cent as reported by Singh and Pant (1998); Das *et al.* (2002).

Inorganic phosphorus is essential for energy transformation at cellular level and normal phospholipids metabolism and it is also an integral part of many coenzymes and its involvement in phospholipids and CAMP synthesis (Seifi *et al.*, 2005). Significantly reductions in fertility and higher number of service per conception had been reported by Morrow (1969) in phosphorus deficient animals. The repeat breeders had significantly lower mean inorganic phosphorus level than that of normal cyclic animals as reported by Das *et al.* (2002) reporting 4.729 ± 0.150 against 5.513± 0.265 mg per cent; Chandrahar *et al.* (2003) reporting 3.98 ± 0.05 against 4.6 ± 0.04 mg per cent and Ceylan *et al.* (2008) reporting 5.19 ± 0.22 against 6.30 ± 0.23 mg per cent. Awasthi and Kharche (1987) reported that the infertile repeat breeder cows had lower (3.73 ± 0.29 mg %) inorganic phosphorus levels than normal cyclic cows (5.06 ± 1.19 mg %) and similar findings was also showed by the author (Table 6). Das *et al.* (2009) also observed that the serum inorganic phosphorus concentration was higher significantly in the animals with normal ovulation (5.45 ± 0.15 mg %) than the animals with anovulation (4.45± 0.14 mg %).

Glucose is the key energy substrate in the bovine ovary, and a sufficient supply of glucose is essential to sustain the ovarian activity as reported by Nishimoto *et al.* (2006). During oestrus if hypoglycaemia occurs then it might lead to lack of energy to spermatozoa, ovum and embryo (McClure, 1968). Chandrahar *et al.* (2003) reported that the blood glucose level might also denote the fertility status of cows. The mean level of serum glucose in repeat breeder crossbred cows at different days of oestrus ranged from 65.69 ± 11.36 to 119.94± 11.59 mg/dl (Talukdar *et al.*, 2015). Shiraz Khan *et al.* (2010) reported that the repeat breeding cows showed significantly higher glucose levels on day 5 of the cycle (50.31 ± 4.19 mg/dl) and day 10 (45.60 ± 6.60 mg/dl), whereas significantly lower level (30.93 ± 4.39 mg/dl) was recorded on day 20 of the oestrous cycle when compared to day 5 and 10 of the cycle. Parmer *et al.* (1986) also stated higher level of glucose during the luteal phase in repeat breeders. This altered level of glucose might be the reason for reduced luteal functions in repeat breeding cows (El- Belely, 1993). The higher blood glucose concentrations directly increased the progesterone production by increasing the pulse and mean concentration of LH (Richards *et al.*, 1989) or indirectly stimulate prolonged progesterone release during early luteal phase by increasing insulin level (Mc Ardle and Holtorf, 1989). Joe Arosh *et al.* (1998) reported that poor energy status in repeat breeders due to hypoglycemia could be the reason for impaired hypothalamic hypophyseal ovarian axis and reduced ovarian activities.

The starting material for the biosynthesis of steroid hormones is cholesterol (Hu *et al.*, 2010). The difference in the level of serum cholesterol might be accredited to several functions like fertility status of the animal, stage of the oestrous cycle and genotype. Several workers reported that serum cholesterol was higher in repeat breeder cows as compared to that in normal cows (Sharma *et al.*, 2003). Singh and Pant (1998) however recorded higher serum cholesterol level of 240.9 ± 11.68 mg% in normal cyclic cows as compared to 125.4 ± 4.03 mg% in the repeat breeders. Singh (2003) found level of serum cholesterol at dioestrus as 135.55 ± 1.81 mg% in crossbred cows beside 125.27 ± 1.75 mg% in local cows.

The minerals also varied in repeat breeder animals and it effect on normal ovulatory mechanism. In a study conducted by Das *et al.* (2009) showed that the concentrations of Calcium (mg %), Inorganic Phosphorus (mg %) and Zinc (ppm) differed significantly among the animals with normal ovulation (9.58 ± 0.49, 5.45 ± 0.15 and 1.78 ± 0.02), anovulation (6.48 ± 0.13, 4.45 ± 0.14 and 0.85 ± 0.03) and delayed ovulation (7.36 ± 0.13, 4.96 ± 0.09 and 1.41 ± 0.04). They also reported that the concentrations of Magnesium (mg %) and Manganese (ppm) were found to be significantly lower in the animals with anovulation (2.64 ± 0.04 and 0.14 ± 0.01) compared to the animals with normal (3.12 ± 0.05 and 28 ± 0.01) and delayed ovulation (2.98 ± 0.06 and 0.23 ± 0.01). Thus the results indicated that Calcium, Inorganic Phosphorus and Zinc are probably crucial for the normal ovulatory process and Magnesium and Manganese below the optimum level might have caused anovulation in crossbred cattle.

Low level of plasma protein causes deficiency of certain amino acids which is required for the biosynthesis of gonadotropins and gonadal hormones (Vohra *et al.*, 1995). In repeat breeding cows, highest level of total protein was recorded by Shiraz Khan *et al.* (2010) on day 5 of the cycle (6.55 ± 0.05 g/dl) which was significantly different from the lowest plasma total protein concentration on day 20 of the cycle (6.32 ± 0.01 g/dl) whereas in normally cycling cows, day 0 showed higher concentration of total protein (6.97 ± 0.14 g/dl) when compared to day 15 of the cycle (6.62 ± 0.15 g/dl). Kaitenbach and Dunn (1980) reported that the progesterone played a regulatory role in the synthesis of specific amino acids. This might be the reason for increased demand for protein and amino acids for GnRH and LH synthesis during early luteal phase of the cycle.

The higher level of albumin in normally cycling cows revealed increased demand for amino acids and protein for the biosynthesis of

GnRH and LH to initiate ovulation and this albumin concentration was lowest on day 15 (2.75 ± 0.11 g/ dl) and highest on day 20 of the cycle (2.95 ± 0.05 g/dl) and there was a significant difference between the albumin concentration on day 15 and day 20 of the cycle in repeat breeding cows (Shiraz Khan *et al.*, 2010). The plasma globulin levels also significantly lower in repeat breeder as comparison with normally cycling cows irrespective of days of the cycle. Significantly higher level of plasma globulin was observed by Shiraz Khan *et al.* (2010) in normally cycling cows on day 0 of the cycle (3.82 ± 0.01 g/dl) in contrast with day 20 of the cycle (3.58 ± 0.11 g/dl) where as in repeat breeding cows, significantly lower level of globulin was observed on day 20 of the cycle (3.37 ± 0.07 g/dl) when compared to day 5 of the cycle (3.70 ± 0.07 g/dl). They suggested that globulin functioning as a carrier protein for copper, altered the biosynthesis of specific coenzymes, thus the steroidogenesis during early luteal phase of the cycle in repeat breeding cows.

Summary

There was change in blood biochemical constituents during different days of estrous cycle in repeat breeder cattle and it might be the cause of repeat breeding in cattle because variations in the level of these elements have been found to be associated with various reproductive disorders.

Table 6. Level of serum calcium, inorganic phosphorus, glucose and cholesterol in repeat breeder and normal cyclic crossbred cows at different days of estrous cycle

Blood biochemical constituents	Different days of estrous cycle (6)				
	Day 0	Day 2	Day 8	Day 14	Day 18
Calcium (mg/ dl) Repeat breeder	10.48 ± 1.24	8.43 ± 1.33	9.33 ± 1.91	9.13 ± 0.88	8.26 ± 0.96
Calcium (mg/ dl) Normal breeder	12.55 ± 2.34	11.28 ± 1.79	10.61 ± 2.32	9.48 ± 1.06	11.32 ± 2.71
Inorganic phosphorus (mg/ dl) Repeat breeder	5.97 ± 0.93	5.02 ± 0.55	4.59 ± 0.33	4.51 ± 0.82	4.40 ± 0.49
Inorganic phosphorus (mg/ dl)Normal breeder	6.01± 0.32	5.14 ± 0.64	5.61 ± 0.91	5.98 ± 0.92	6.72 ± 1.02
Glucose (mg/ dl) Repeat breeder	107.31 ± 14.79	77.33 ± 12.57	81.22 ± 14.02	118.14 ± 15.94	119.54 ± 18.45
Glucose (mg/ dl) Normal breeder	108.47 ± 16.20	78.27 ± 2.28	60.72 ± 1.12	89.41 ± 10.47	119.62 ± 25.32
Cholesterol (mg/ dl) Repeat breeder	110.09 ± 13.12	132.03 ± 26.06	118.44 ± 11.44	119.45 ± 12.12	117.09 ± 12.1
Cholesterol (mg/ dl) Normal breeder	120.80 ± 8.43	133.22 ± 13.31	123.93 ± 10.29	124.14 ± 9.72	145.40 ± 20.44

Figures in the parentheses indicate number of animals.

❑❑❑

Chapter-7

Hormonal Profile of Repeat Breeder Dairy Cattle

The major of embryonic loss in dairy cattle occurs in pre implantation stage *i.e* during the first 20 days of pregnancy, when 75-80% of fertilized eggs are lost (Sreenan *et al.*, 1996). One of the causes of embryonic loss is thought to be the inadequate luteal function (Willard *et al.,* 2003). Early embryonic death is one of the causes of repeat breeding in cows. The incidence of repeat breeding, a major factor involved in reduced fertility, varies, ranging from 18 to 24% (Stevenson *et al.*, 1990). About 40% of the repeat-breeding (RB) in cows is due to early embryonic losses (Thatcher *et al.*, 1994). The participation of progesterone (P4) in the upholding of pregnancy and regulation of uterine PGF2á secretion is well recognized (Royal *et al.*, 2000; Lucy, 2001). Progesterone stimulates endometrial gland growth and prepares the uterus to receive and nourish a new embryo. Inadequate luteal progesterone has been concerned as a cause for abnormal embryonic development and early embryonic loss (Ahmad *et al.,* 1996). The repeat breeder cows have lower progesterone concentrations than cows with normal fertility during the first week after ovulation (Kimura *et al.*, 1987). Mann and Lamming (1995) found that cows with low progesterone concentrations during the luteal phase of the estrous cycle had an enhanced surge of PGF2á after oxytocin treatment on days 15 and 16 of the cycle. The period during embryonic growth and differentiation are highly dependent on uterine secretions. As a result, delayed embryonic development in RB cows may be related to insufficient progesterone secretion during the first week post insemination. The late embryo development may impair maternal recognition of pregnancy since the embryo will not be able to produce sufficient quantities of interferon [tau] to prevent PGF2á secretion and luteolysis occurs (Mann and Lamming, 1995).

In a study Gupta *et al.* (1998) observed that the mean blood serum progesterone levels on the day of oestrus were 0.29 ng/ml in the cows that conceived and 0.32 ng/ml in those not conceiving. They also reported that on the day 18th post- insemination the progesterone level was significantly higher (6.29 ng/ml) in blood serum in the cows that conceived than in the cows which did not conceive (1.11 ng/ml). Hafez (1987) who stated that level of progesterone in cows with 21 day cycle increased rapidly from day 3 to day 8 of oestrus with a much slower rate of increase from day 8 through day 17. Low progesterone concentrations during an oestrous cycle lead to delay stimulatory effect on uterine responsiveness to oxytocin during the late luteal phase of the subsequent cycle resulting increase in PGF(2alpha) secretion which might interfere with luteal maintenance during the early stages of pregnancy (Shaham-Albalancy *et al.*, 2001). The lower mean concentration of serum progesterone on day 0, 4, 11and 16 of oestrus as 0.40 ± 0.03, 0.78 ± 0.05, 2.25 ± 0.20 and 2.82 ± 0.26 ng/ml respectively in normal breeding cows and 0.46 ± 0.08, 0.72 ± 0.12, 2.04 ± 0.23 and 2.49 ± 0.33 ng/ml respectively in repeat breeding cows as recorded by Shukla *et al.* (2000). Venkatesan *et al.* (2005) reported that the level of serum progesterone on 0 day of oestrus (0.558 ± 0.001 ng/ml) was found to be higher in repeat breeding cows than in regular breeding cows (0.1922 ± 0.077 ng/ml). They also stated that the serum progesterone level on day 7 was lower in repeat breeding cows (1.0147 ± 0.457 ng/ml) than in regular breeding cows (3.151 ± 0.092 ng/ml). On the other hand Dhami *et al.* (2009) reported that the average serum progesterone concentration of repeat breeders was significantly lower than that of normal cyclic cows (2.75 ± 0.54 and 3.87 ± 1.05 ng/ml respectively).

The level of serum estradiol 17-β is higher during oestrus and towards the prooestrus (18 day of oestrus) and lower on day 8 of oestrus. A high amount of estrogen, interestingly, has an opposite stimulatory effect on the gonadotropins. LH and FSH begin to increase in high fashion. As more estrogen is secreted, more LH receptors are made by the theca cells, inciting theca cells to create more androgen that will become estrogen downstream. This positive feedback loop causes LH to spike sharply, and it is this spike that causes ovulation. Following ovulation, LH stimulates the formation of the corpus luteum. Estrogen has since dropped to negative stimulatory levels after ovulation and therefore serves to maintain the concentration of FSH and LH. Shukla *et al.* (2000) reported that on day 0, 4, 11 and 16; the mean values as 20.25 ± 0.70, 11.20 ± 0.84, 7.71 ± 1.49 and 6.56 ± 1.31 pg/ml respectively in normal breeding cows and 20.93 ± 1.14, 13.08 ± 0.98, 8.60 ± 1.31 and 9.39 ± 0.88 pg/ml respectively in repeat breeding cows. Venkatesan *et al.* (2005) recorded the level of serum estrogen on 0 day of oestrus in regular and repeat breeder cows as 7.201 ± 1.29 and 6.212 ± 0.216 pg/ml and on day 7 the values were 2.99 ± 0.05 and 2.104 ± 0.012 pg/ml in regular breeding and repeat breeding cows respectively. The level of serum estradiol 17- ß concentration on day of oestrus as 13.2 pg/ml in animals which conceived following insemination and 13.5 pg/ml in animals which failed to conceive as reported by Gupta *et al.* (1998).

Summary

There was change in hormonal level during different days of estrous cycle in repeat breeder cattle (Table 7) which is below from the normal cyclic cow. The oestradiol generally exerts a positive feedback on the hypothalamus and pituitary gland, which increases the frequency of the GnRH pulses. Above a certain threshold level of oestradiol, the hypothalamus responds with a surge of GnRH which in turn, induces an LH surge that initiates ovulation. So, if the level of oestradiol is less, it hampers the normal physiological function and ultimately it associated with reproductive malfunction and repeat breeding. On the other hand, progesterone stimulates endometrial gland growth and prepares the uterus to accept and nurture a new embryo. Inadequate luteal progesterone as we have seen in repeat breeder has been concerned as a cause for abnormal embryonic development and early embryonic loss which might be responsible for repeat breeding.

Table 7. Level of serum estradiol 17-β and progesterone (Mean ± SE) in repeat breeder and normal cyclic crossbred cows at different days of oestrous cycle.

Different days of oestrous cycle	Estradiol 17-β (pg/ml) in repeat breeder (6)	Estradiol 17-β (pg/ml) in normal breeder (6)	Progesterone (ng/ml) in repeat breeder (6)	Progesterone (ng/ml) in normal breeder (6)
0	$8.92_{a} \pm 0.85$	$10.13_{a} \pm 1.32$	$0.6^{a} \pm 0.05$	$0.98^{a} \pm 0.27$
2	$7.92_{a} \pm 0.8$	$7.02_{bc} \pm 0.71$	$0.53^{a} \pm 0.09$	$2.17^{a} \pm 1.45$
8	$2.21_{b} \pm 0.04$	$4.39_{c} \pm 0.63$	$3.64^{b} \pm 1.03$	$10.56^{ab} \pm 2.61$
14	$4.75_{a} \pm 1.85$	$6.46_{bc} \pm 0.33$	$8.24^{b} \pm 2.59$	$11.56^{b} \pm 2.45$
18	$6.34_{a} \pm 0.91$	$7.97_{ac} \pm 0.64$	$1.2^{b} \pm 0.49$	$8.32^{a} \pm 2.65$

Figures in the parentheses indicate number of animals.

Means bearing similar subscript and superscript in a column do not differ significantly.

❑❑❑

Chapter-8

Diagnosis of Various Reproductive Disorders Responsible for Repeat Breeding Syndrome

Diagnosing the cause of repeat breeding in dairy cattle is often extremely difficult and evaluations are concerned with the health of the animal as well as the condition of the genital tract, the physiological functioning of the ovaries and consecutive growth and development of the fertilised embryo. Many diagnostic tools are available; it is usually difficult to get a correct diagnostic because sometimes it is unprofitable.

For primary evaluation, a complete clinical history should be obtained at herd and individual level. The history regarding age, parity, milk yield, previous diseases, reproductive indexes, oestrous cycles', characteristics, oestrus behaviour, insemination schedule, insemination technique, bulls and its semen quality, oestrus detection technique, blood biochemical and hormonal status, food and farm hygiene should be registered first. The reproductive status of animals must be evaluated according to their production. The vulva, vagina, cervix, uterus, fallopian tubes and ovaries must be examined to diagnoses of reproductive defects.

1. Clinico-gynaecological examination

The physical examination is important to identify congenital or acquired anatomical defects such as pneumovagina, vulvar defects, tumors or injuries. The anatomical shape, size and location of the genital tract, its secretions around vulva or tail should be evaluated. The vaginal contents should be examined to detect urine (if urovagina), pus (if endometritis, vaginitis; Figure 8), blood (post-ovulation or some diseases) or clear and clean mucus (associated with heat).

Vaginoscopy with vaginal speculum is helpful to visualize the vaginal cavity and cervix. The faeces should be removed from the rectum and the perineal area, vestibule and clitoral fossa should be cleaned. The vaginal speculum which must be clean, dry, sterile, and lubricated- is inserted in direction of the pelvic canal. Once it crossed the vestibule, the negative pressure inside allows air to penetrate. Hyperemia may result in 30-60 sec, which hampers the assessment of the vaginal mucosa coloration. The vestibule which acts as a defensive barrier of the female genital tract hinders the entry of the speculum. If this does not occur, dysfunctions can be present (e.g. pneumovagina). Such examination can also be help in diagnosing cervicitis or vaginitis (Sah and Nakao, 2006) or changes in cervical morphology (Modi *et al.*, 2011) which could be a possible cause of repeat breeding especially in natural mating. The anatomic anomalies such as kinked cervix (Modi *et al.*, 2011) which can affect fertility can be identified with transrectal palpations and vaginoscopic examinations. Similarly, if any material is accumulated into the vagina, speculum helps to localize its origin and also helps in further laboratory examination.

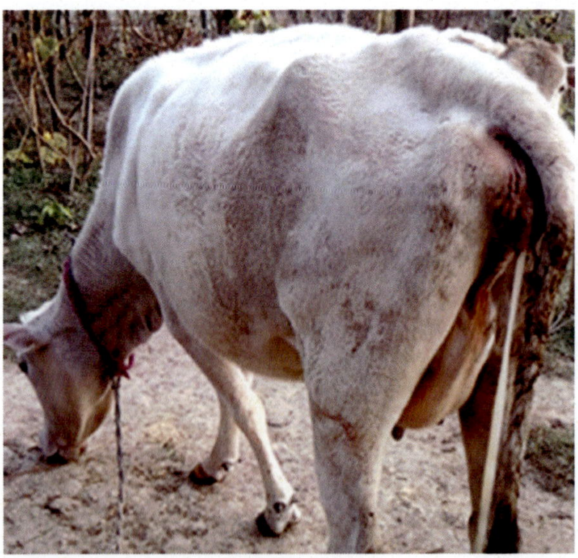

Figure 8. Dirty uterine discharge indicates uterine infection

2. Per rectal examination

Per rectal examination is a widely used diagnostic method in cattle with high accuracy, it is easy to be implemented and at low cost in comparison with other sophisticated techniques (Figure 9). Rubber or Plastic gloves are lubricated and then faeces are withdrawn. Air should not be entered into the rectum to get a more relaxed mucosa and easily manipulate the structures beneath. The cervix is accessible as a solid structure, tubular, fibrous, with 3-4 folds projected inside and localized on pelvic floor in normal non-pregnant cows. It is cylindrical, with a length of 5-10 cm and a diameter of 1.5-7.0 cm. The uterus can be palpated cranially. During estrus, the uterus become turgid, erect and coiled. During luteal phase though it is soft and flaccid but palpation is a bit more difficult; it is a consequence of the progesterone action, released from CL. This palpation helps to diagnose anomalies such as kinked cervix, uterine infections. After that, one should proceed towards the ovaries. The ovaries are located ventrolaterally to the pelvis floor, and sometimes placed under the bone. During anestrus, ovary size ranges from 2 to 3 cm approximately. Follicles (at different stages of growth) and CLs (hemorrhagic, mature or/and albicans) are developed at the ovaries and its size could suggest some diseases as well as its presence/absence also denotes the hormonal status of the animals. The repeat breeder cows are diagnosed to be affected with anovulation when per rectum examination of the ovaries contain tensed follicles and not ovulating till 24 hours of oestrus and also did not reveal formation of corpus luteum even on day 8 of oestrus. A cow diagnosed to be affected with delayed ovulation when rectal palpation of the ovaries indicated presence of Graafian follicle on one of the ovaries till day 2 of oestrus but a mature corpus luteum on day 8. Cows under normal ovulation category revealed formation of corpus haemorrhagicum within day 2 of oestrous and without any detectable genital abnormalities but they repeating due to some managemental error. Repeat breeder cows showing mucopurulent discharge during rectal examination on day 0 were considered as repeat breeder cows with uterine infection. Physical examination of cervico-vaginal mucus is often the first diagnostic method of finding infection in the genital tract of the cows.

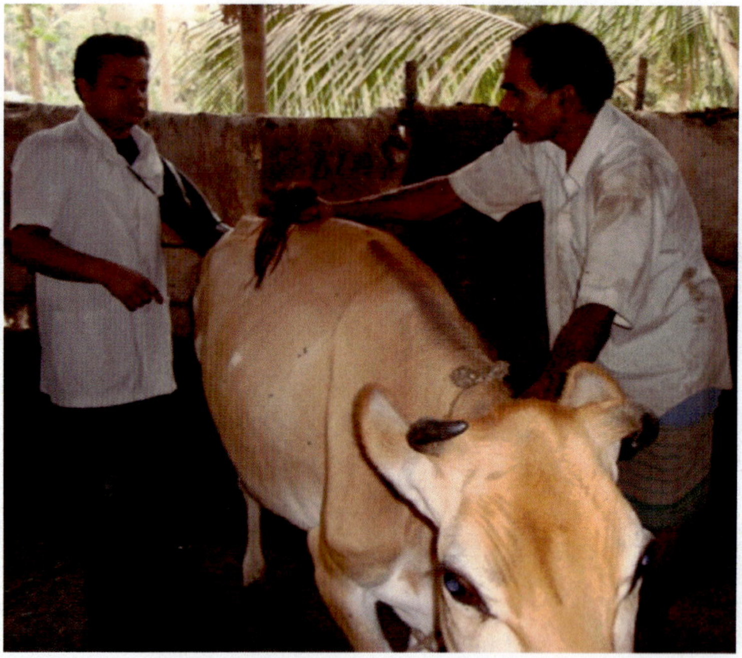

Figure 9. Per rectal examination of the animal

3. Ultrasonography (USG)

The first concept of ultrasound came in the year 1877 with the discovery of piezoelectricity by French physicist Pierre Curie. Thirty-five years later, sonographic imaging was developed by French professor and physicist Paul Langevin. In addition, Dr. Karl Theodore Dussik of Austria published the first paper on medical ultrasonics in 1942, based on his research on transmission ultrasound investigation of the brain; and Professor Ian Donald of Scotland developed practical technology and applications for ultrasound in the 1950's. The real-time ultrasound was first conducted and demonstrated by Chaffeux *et al.* (1982) in pregnant cattle. Later, the ultrasound images of normal ovarian structures showed by Pierson & Ginther (1984) in superovulated heifers. Reeves *et al.* (1984) demonstrated the echogenicity of the cystic CL. By using transrectal ultrasonic technology we should enhanced our ability to assess the reproductive organs in cattle and to follow the dynamic interactions between ovarian follicular cohorts. The 2-3 mm follicles can also be seen, quantified and sequentially monitored. The practical utility of ultrasound in reproduction include routine assessment of follicular and luteal development, and differential diagnosis of cystic ovaries

(Rajamahendran, 1994), ovarian abscesses and tumors, which can be considered factors associated with RBC syndrome. The real-time ultrasonography helps to evaluate the uterus by detecting changes in shape and echotexture related with circulating hormone concentrations during the oestrous cycle, and thereby detecting hormonal imbalances. It is also helps for diagnosis of different pathological conditions of the female reproductive tract such as metritis, pyometra, maceration or mummification. The ultrasonic diagnostic features of endometritis include increased endometrial thickness and increased intraluminal uterine fluid accumulation (Tandle and Purohit, 2013). The real time ultrasonography has also proven to be a valuable tool for diagnosing pregnancy and assessing fetal viability (Yeager *et al.*, 1992). In addition the ovarian blood flow that can be helpful in predicting embryonic mortality can be gained by colour Doppler ultrasonography (Honparkhe *et al.*, 2004). By using the technique of hysteroscopy, (Purohit *et al.*, 2013) we can gain additional information about the uterine lumen such as hemorrhages which is not detectable by ultrasonography. The timing of ovulation can be monitored by frequent ultrasonographic examinations (6–12 h after estrus) and visualization of the disruption of ovulatory follicle (Purohit, 2008) can helps in fix time A.I. The delayed and anovulatory oestrus can be more efficiently determined by ultrasonographic examination with formation of corpus luteum on day 5 post estrus (Neglia *et al.*, 2015). The early embryonic deaths can be evaluated by using sequential transrectal ultrasonography (Awasthi *et al.*, 2007) and the disappearance of a previously visible gestational sac/fetus and/or fluids suggest embryonic death. Such evaluations are very difficult with per rectal palpations as most bubaline embryonic deaths occur between days 25–45 (Awasthi *et al.*, 2007).

4. Hormonal function test

The gonadotropic hormones, neurotransmitters and other substances are involved in the regulation of the reproductive cycle in cow. Its synthesis, release, action or interaction, imbalance could be related to reproductive alterations as repeat estrus and reduced fertility.

Progesterone can be considered as a key hormone for the reproductive capacity. Low progesterone concentrations during an oestrous cycle had been reported to a delayed stimulatory effect on uterine responsiveness to oxytocin during the late luteal phase of the subsequent cycle resulting increase in $PGF_2\alpha$ secretion which may interfere with luteal maintenance during the early stages of pregnancy (Shaham-Albalancy *et al.*, 2001). Therefore progesterone assay is an objective and accurate test to determine the ovarian function and to diagnose certain diseases that otherwise could not be correctly evaluated, such as delayed ovulation, persistent luteal activity, ovarian cysts or suprabasal progesterone levels (Waldmann *et al.*, 2000). This assessment during estrus, could confirm that the hormonal environment is within the correct hormonal framework. Then, estimation in an around day 19-21 after AI, it could be an effective method to detect females with pregnancy failure. Because the level of progesterone in cows with 21 day cycle increased rapidly from day 3 to day 8 of oestrus with a much slower rate of increase from day 8 through day 17 (Talukdar, 2010) while on the day 18th of post-insemination the progesterone level was significantly higher (Gupta *et al.*, 1998) in blood serum in the cows that conceived. Generally radioimmunoassay (RIA) and enzyme immunoassay (ELISA) are the usual analytical techniques for determining steroids in biological fluids.

5. Oviductal patency test

The oviductal permeability and its determination is interesting, although it is difficult to carry out. The injection of 500 ml of sterile solution containing 30 gm of starch has been described by Kessy & Noakes (1979). It is injected intraperitoneally and the starch reaches the oviduct and descends to the cervical mucus if the fallopian tubes are permeable which takes about 12 hours to arrive at the cervical mucus, where it will remain between 2 and 4 days. Then a sample of mucus is collected, stained with lugol and observed under the microscope. Other test to study the oviductal patency is the PSP dye test (Phenol sulphonapthalein Dye Test) where phenol sulphonfthalein is infused into the uterine horn (Kothari *et al.*, 1978). In this test a Foley catheter is inserted through the uterus and the balloon is inflated on the end of the horn before dye is infused. If the oviduct is normal, the dye will cross it, reach the abdominal cavity, and is eliminated by urine. Bladder is catheterized 20 minutes later and urine turns to reddish if oviduct is normal. After 4 hours, the test can be repeated in the other oviduct (Figure 10). In addition of this, another diagnostic technique to check the oviductal patency is the collecting oocytes or embryos, either with or without superovulation treatments. If they are collected, it is possible to transfer them to cows without reproductive problems, in which case it also becomes a therapeutic tool to overcome this syndrome.

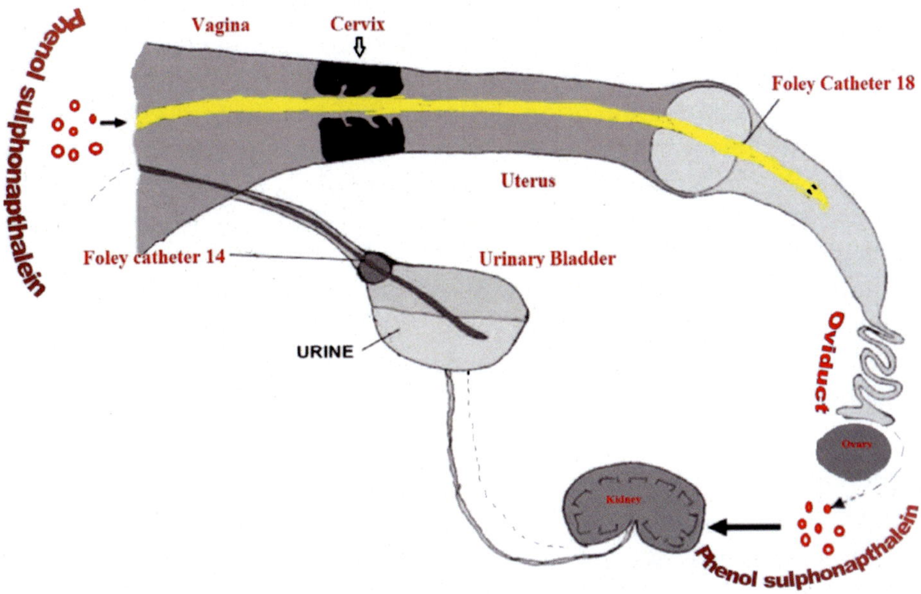

Figure 10. Phenol sulphonapthalein Dye Test for evaluation of oviductal patency

6. Endometrial cytology and uterine bacterial culture

A plenty of pathogens could be localized at the female reproductive tract, affecting the success of fertilization. The infectious diseases could aggravate vulvitis, vaginitis, cervicitis or endometritis, and it is important to diagnose these disorders. Generally, the inflammation begins with bacterial contamination into the uterine lumen, and continues with adhesion of pathogens to the mucosa, colonization or penetration of the epithelium, and/or release of endotoxins. These uterine inflammations, even in the absence of active bacterial infection, may disrupt embryonic survival and incite RBC syndrome. The endometrial bacteriological examination is important to detect pathogens implicated in infertility. In cattle, the samples can be taken using a catheter connected to a syringe containing 30-60 ml of sterile saline. It is deposited into the uterus and then it is removed and cultured. The clinical or subclinical endometritis could be diagnosed. The endometrial cytology is a realistic technique to diagnose subclinical endometritis, when clinical signs are absent. The presence of neutrophils and its number indicates the type and grade of endometrial inflammation. Another field test is available to detect the subclinical endometritis *i.e.* White side test. The original test was described by Whiteside (1939) and was modified by Schalm *et al.*, (1971). In this test where cervico-vaginal mucus is collected aseptically using the sterile A.I. sheath with a syringe. Then 1-2 ml of cervico-vaginal mucus and equal quantity (1-2 ml) of test reagent (5% Sodium hydrooxide) taken in a test tube and mix it gently. After mixing, the test tube should be heated up to the boiling point and then allow it to cool for some time. After that observe the changes in intensity of the color in the test tube and interpret accordingly. The development of color *i.e.* light yellow to dark yellow in the test sample after boiling is considered as positive for uterine infection (Figure 11).

Color intensity	Grades of uterine infection
No color	0 (Normal)
Light yellow	+ (Mild)
Yellow	++ (Moderate)
Dark Yellow	+++ (Severe)

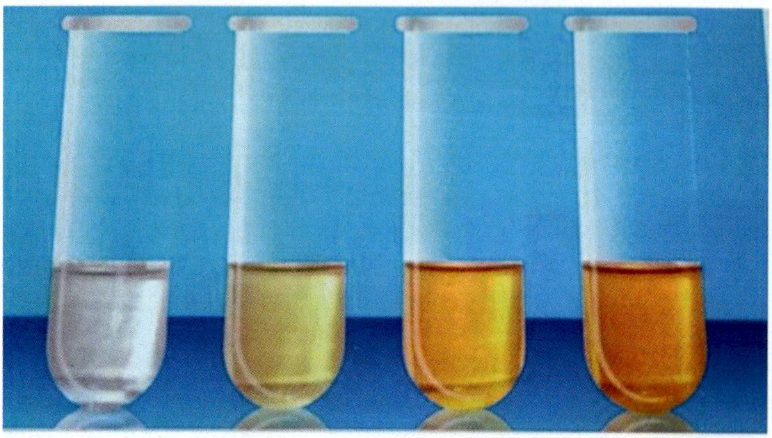

Figure 11. Color intensity after White side test

7. Level of oxidant and antioxidant markers

The oxidant/antioxidant markers in repeat breeding cows' serum have shown increased malondialdehyde (MDA) and nitric oxide (NO) and decreased catalase (CAT), superoxide dismutase (SOD), ascorbic acid (ASCA), reduced glutathione (GSH-R) and total antioxidant capacity (TAC) (Ahmed *et al.*, 2010). Everyone knows that in a healthy body, reactive oxygen species (ROS) and antioxidants remain in balance. When this balance is disrupted towards an over abundance of ROS, oxidative stress (OS) occurs. Also, the ROS have a important role in pathological processes involving the female reproductive tract, and it affect multiple physiological processes from oocyte maturation to fertilization, embryo development and pregnancy (Kumar *et al.,* 2012). The repeat breeder cows showed increased MDA and NO and decreased CAT, SOD, ASCA, GSH-R and TAC (Hanafi *et al.,* 2008). The use of these markers in repeat breeding cattle is currently limited.

8. Serum biochemical profile

The variations in circulating levels of biochemicals have been recorded in repeat breeding cattle (as discussed in chapter no. 6) however, using serum biochemical profile or trace mineral status to predict potential fertility is far from perfect (Purohit, 2008) and such evaluations can possibly be used to predict deficiencies in representative samples from large herds.

Summary

Diagnosing the cause of repeat breeding in individual cows is often extremely difficult and evaluations are oriented towards evaluating the health of the genital tract, physiological functioning of the ovaries and sequential growth and development of the embryo. A combination of imaging techniques, visual estimates, and perrectal examination is suggested by various workers. The advanced imaging techniques such as ultrasonography, endoscopy, metabolic profiles, uterine biopsies and tubal patency testing etc. are helps in easy and early diagnosis of the various causes of repeat breeding which will be help for easy therapeutic management as well as success rate will also be increased.

Chapter-9

Therapeutic Efficacy of Different Treatment Protocols for Repeat Breeding Syndrome

The specific therapeutic management for repeat breeding will depend on the underlying cause or causes. Due to the number of different causes, the treatments is also varies. Therefore before treating the repeat breeder cow, a thorough investigation is required. Here some of the treatment protocol is discussed.

1. Manual induction of ovulation at anovulatory oestrus

In this technique the Graafian follicle was manually ruptured between day 1 and day 2 of oestrus. To rupture the Graafian follicle, the ovary should be lifted in between the index and middle fingers and gentle pressure was exerted at the base of fluctuating area with the help of the tip of the thumb. The pressure should be released as soon as the follicle is ruptured (Figure 12). Van Rensburg and De Vos (1962) in their classic study observed that only one cow out of 36 conceived when Graafian follicle was manually ruptured at the time of A.I. Deka (1994) also recorded 54.54 per cent conception rate in anovulatory repeat breeder crossbred cows by inducing ovulation mechanically during late oestrus and inseminating the cows normally in the subsequent oestrus. Sixty per cent of conception rate was recorded by Das *et al.* (2002) in repeat breeder cows with A.I. at late hours of oestrus following rupture of Graafian follicle. Talukdar (2010) recorded 100 per cent conception rate by rupturing the Graafian follicle manually and A.I. at subsequent oestrus in the anovulatory repeat breeder cow. This finding clearly indicated that all the anovulatory cows ovulated normally in the subsequent oestrous cycle. The normal ovulation obtaining in the subsequent cycle might be attributed to the measurable amount of progesterone secreted from the regressing corpus luteum of the previous cycle which might have helped in final growth and maturation of the follicles and caused their successful ovulation in the next cycle (Van Rensburg and De Vos, 1962). El-Belely (1993) also reported that a small amount of progesterone injected during early oestrus could hasten ovulation.

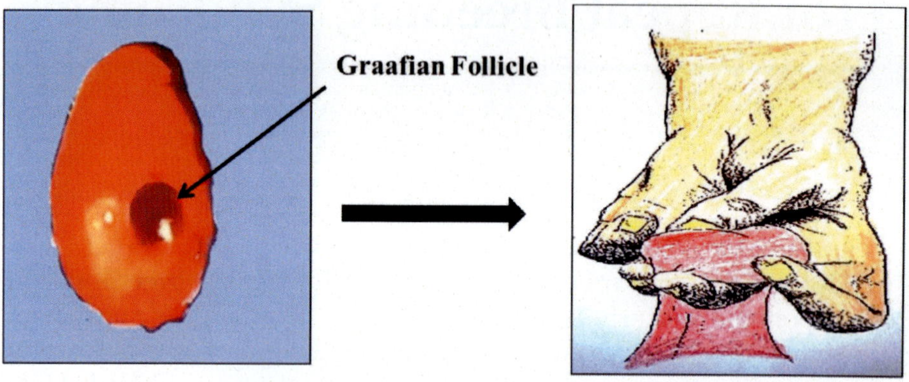

Figure 12. Technique of manual rupture of the Graafian follicle

2. Ovulation induced by Human Chorionic Gonadotropin (hCG) hormone

According to Roberts (1971) intravenous administration of 2000-5000 IU of chorionic gonadotropin hastened or promoted ovulation in cows. Zemjanis (1980) stated that the intravenous administration of 1000 to 2500 IU of hCG or of a comparable dose of other LH acting hormone preparation could be used in the treatment of anovulation in cows. The highest conception rate of 83.33 % per cent was recorded by Chaudhary *et al.* (2009) in repeat breeder cows using 1500 IU of hCG intravenously on day 4 post breeding. Das (2002) in his experiment on repeat breeding crossbred cows recorded 66.67 and 50.00 per cent conception rates in cows with anovulation and delayed ovulation respectively by using 1500 IU of hCG intravenously immediately following artificial insemination. Talukdar *et al.* (2013) recorded that 100 per cent conception rate when the anovulatory repeat breeders were treated with 3000 IU of hCG.

3. Multiple Artificial Inseminations during Spontaneous Oestrus

In ensuring fertilisation, the importance of AI timing with respect to ovulation has repeatedly been emphasized. Inseminations early in oestrus yield low pregnancy rates either due to fertilization failure or due to early embryonic mortality (Singh *et al.*, 2005). Despite a well timed (in respect to onset of oestrus) single AI in repeat breeder leads to lower pregnancy rate compared with controls (Singh *et al.*, 2005). When delayed ovulation occurs, it may lead to poor tubal milieu and altered contractility compromises sperm survival and impairs proper gamete transport. Under these grounds, re-inseminations during oestrus have been found to only marginally improve fertility in spontaneous repeat-breeder animals. The problem in Repeat breeder might be alleviated if high numbers of fertilisable spermatozoa are available at the time of ovulation. A single second AI, in repeat-breeding animals, has led to an improvement in pregnancy rates and Stevenson *et al.* (1990) reported a marginal increase in pregnancy rate from 32.1% to 33.5% when a single second AI was performed 12 to 16 h after first AI. Albihn (1991) has reported an increase in pregnancy rate from 9.5% to 52.9%, in cows that ovulated 24 h after first AI, when a single second AI was performed 24 h (re-insemination close to ovulation) after first AI. Improvement of pregnancy rate following re-inseminations in repeat-breeding animals should therefore not be disregarded. It may be speculated that AI closer to ovulation may provide more spermatozoa with high fertilizing capacity at the site of fertilization and thus lead to improved conception rates. A possible reason for this improvement could be the shorter exposure to an adverse maternal milieu before they attempt fertilization.

4. Treatment with Gonadotropin-releasing hormone (GnRH)

Several different strategies for RBS treatment have been reported. A gonadotropin-releasing hormone (GnRH) application significantly increases the conception rate in repeat breeders. On the other hand, that frequent insemination (every 6 hrs) can also increase the conception rate in cases of RBS. However, no significant results were found by double (repeated) insemination of cows within 12 or 18 hrs without an application of GnRH. Shahneh *et al.* (2008) indicated that the injection of GnRH at the time of insemination increased ovulation (65% vs 47.5%) as well as conception rates (55% vs 25%) in repeat breeder cow. Yildiz *et al.* (2009) reported that the pregnancy rates in repeat breeder cows treated with 10.5 ìg GnRH on day 12 post mating were higher (77.7% vs 50.00%) than those in the saline treated control group. They also recommended that pregnancy rates should increased in repeat breeder cow following the treatment with GnRH on 11-12 days post-mating.

5. Treatment with exogenous progesterone

Progesterone is secreted by the corpora lutea which suppresses the further development of follicles and the secretion of estrogen. High levels of progesterone and low levels of estrogen will stop a cow from coming into heat. Progesterone is essential for preparing the uterus to receive the fertilized egg and maintains the proper uterine environment for continuation of pregnancy. Estrogen and progesterone are not completely separate in their functions since both must be present for certain processes to take place. This estrogen/ progesterone concentration ratio dictates the onset and duration of behavioral estrus. Development of the uterus is initiated by estrogen and completed by progesterone. Estrogen causes contraction of the uterus near the time of estrus and ovulation, which help in sperm transport. Progesterone has a quieting effect on the uterus so that there are no contractions which might disturb pregnancy. Das *et al.* (2002) treated the repeat breeding cows with anovulation and delayed ovulation with two intramuscular injection of 500 mg progesterone (Duraprogen), one immediately after A.I. and the other 4 days after A.I. and obtained 60% conception rate. Awasthi *et al.* (2002) treated the repeat breeder cows with single intramuscular dose of 500 mg of hydroxy progesterone caproate, between day 6 to 8 post insemination, and found significantly higher conception rate in the treated cows as compared to control cows. Chaudhary *et al.* (2009) treated the repeat breeder cows with 500 mg of hydroxy progesterone caproate (Dinolutin) intramuscularly on day 4 post breeding and found 83.33 % conception rate. Talukdar *et al.* (2013) recorded that 100 per cent conception rate by treating the repeat breeder cows with 750 mg of progesterone intramuscularly on 3rd, 10th and 17th day of A.I.

6. Treatment of Repeat Breeding in Dairy Cows with Lugol's Iodine

The repeat breeder cows sometimes got infected and their repeat breeding is judged as subclinical endometritis (Grohan and Saoloemi,

1995) which leads to silent heat, failure of inseminations and repeat breeding in dairy cows. The repeat breeding syndrome also be due to trace elements deficiencies particularly iodine deficiency. The iodine is essential for initiation of follicular wave dynamic, ovarian activities, release of best quality mature oocytes and improvement of rate of service per conception in dairy cows (Sarkar, 2006). The iodine while infused in the uterus could be absorbed from the genital tract, transferred to the thyroid gland and associated with thyroid binding globulin (TBG) in the thyroid gland to produce thyroxin (Yu and Tak-yin, 1993). However, the Lugol's iodine has a broad spectrum bactericidal, fungicidal anti protozoa effect (Sheldon *et al.*, 2006). These activities of iodine will enhance the healing of the endometrium to restore its activities. Also, the internal cellular metabolism of the reproductive system including the ovaries will also be improved by infusion of diluted Lugol's iodine (Sarkar, 2006). The diluted Lugol's iodine infusion into the uterus of the repeat breeder dairy cows at pre-servicing improved the conception rate and reduced the length of the days open. This could be due to the potent bactericidal effects of the solution, adjustment of the reproductive tract pH before servicing, the slight hyperemia of the endometrium which enhanced uterine blood circulation and increased the defence mechanisms of the reproductive system that become reasonably efficient (Sarkar, 2006). The infusion of diluted Lugol's iodine into the uterus at post-servicing of the repeat breeder dairy cows had less effect on the rate of service per conception and the days open. The difference between these two is definitely due to sub-clinical endometritis which disturbs the uterine pH and decreases the lively hood of the sperms.

7. Nutritional treatments

The deficiencies of various nutritional components have been described as causes of repeat breeding. The ration provided to the animal containing higher concentration of inorganic iodine from 8-12 days before estrus improve the stimulation of the pituitary gland (McDonald *et al.*, 1961). The repeat breeder cows should supplement with copper and magnesium, to minimizing the fertility problems (Ingraham *et al.*, 1987). The deficiencies of these minerals have been associated with infertility, anemia or immune suppression. The ratio of these minerals can be modified in the ration according to season or agriculture practices, or as a consequence of mineral availability alteration associated with some dietary components (e.g. diets containing high level of protein reduce the copper plasma concentration). It has recently been investigated that beta-carotene, precursor of vitamin A, involved in the formation and function of Corpus Luteum, as it is improves the progesterone synthesis and reduces the luteal hypofunction (Wang *et al.*, 1988). The deficiencies of phosphorus and zinc are responsible for low levels of progesterone production, which could be the cause of failures in fertilization or early embryonic death. The unsaturated fatty acid diets not only improve the milk yield but also increases the embryo development rates when administered at dry and postpartum periods.

8. Assisted reproductive techniques

The unusual implantation and transport of gametes are associated with endometrial defects, resulting repeat breeding. The assisted reproductive techniques, such as in vitro production of embryos and intraperitoneal insemination (Figure 13), have been projected to solve this problem. Intraperitoneal insemination could be an alternative procedure to the normal deposition of semen in the genital tract of the cow (Lopez-Gatius, 1995). It is considered that the uterine infection is also responsible for conception failure which may lead to repeat breeding and it is often difficult to detect in field conditions if it is subclinical. Therefore a bypass from vagina to peritoneal area (around the ovary) is possible to avoid the negative effects of altered uterine environment on the sperm quality. It has been noticed that the majority of embryonic abnormalities occurs in the oviducts, but are not apparent until 6-7 days of post-breeding (Tanaka *et al.,* 1994). Therefore, the oocytes of repeat breeders are competent to reach the blastocyst stage. IVM, IVF and ET techniques are helpful to improve the reproductive success in these animals.

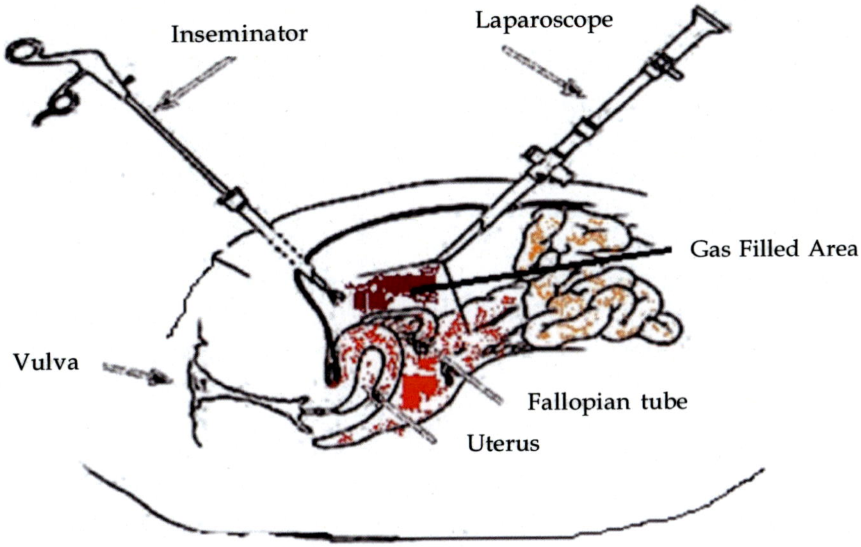

Figure 13. Method of intraperitoneal insemination

9. Intrauterine therapy

The reproductive tract infections which may be lead to repeat breeding syndrome is very often overlooked by clinicians. As a prophylactic measures, the uterine administration of either antiseptic or antibiotic solutions 24 hrs after mating/AI, helps to improve fertility (Tanaka *et al.*, 1994). The studies on bacteriology and histology of the uterus suggested that the non-specific genital infection is one of the main causes of repeat breeding, and it is concluded that the antimicrobial treatments (chloramphenicol, gentamicin, enrofloxacin, tetracycline, ciprofloxacin etc.) could improve the reproductive performance of the animals (Santana *et al.*, 1998).

10. Aquapuncture, as an alternative medicinal therapy for Repeat Breeding Syndrome

Acupuncture is a very old technique; where fish and bone needles may have first been used in China approximately 3000 years ago. Acupuncture typically refers to the use of needles alone (dry needles). The points of acupuncture typically communicate with points where small nerve bundles penetrate the fascia, are close to nerves, or close to blood vessels which have their own innervations or motor points in muscle (Hwang and Egerbacher, 2001). The TCM meridians or channels often follow the propagated sensation along a nerve, and some may follow lymphatic channels (Hwang and Egerbacher, 2001). Regrettably, there is a shortage of scientific study published on use of acupuncture in reproduction, particularly in the English language. Earlier studies suggest that the neuropeptides released due to acupuncture stimulation may act on gonadotropin releasing hormone (GnRH) (Stener-Victorin *et al.*, 1996). The utility of some alternative medicines, such as moxibustion, has also been established to reduce the incidence of repeat breeding syndrome (Hosaha and Nakama, 2002). The moxas (balls of about 3 cm in diameter) containing 2 g of *Artemisia* spp. are applied on nine points of the skin and burned for 15 min. The therapy are used for 3 consecutive days, and then repeated during the heat. Hosaha and Nakama (2002) described that an increase in blood flow at the uterine arteries, which is considered to improve fertility. In a study, Lin *et al.* (2002) treated the repeat breeder cows with simple aquapuncture therapy (acupuncture combined with injection). They treated two dairy herds (one in Hsinchu County and the other in Tainan County). Both herds they had used gonadotropin-releasing hormone (GnRH) before to treat the symptom but the success rate was poor—about 30%. Therefore, the cows that failed to respond to GnRH, they used the aquapuncture treatment. They had 18 animals (two heifers and 16 cows) that had failed to conceive to 3-9 services were treated by aquapuncture, in which 10 ml and 5 ml of 50% glucose solution were injected at the depression in the center of the lumbo sacral space) and at Kidney Shelf, the depression in the space between the lumbar vertebral transverse processes 5-6) acupoints, respectively with a 21G, 1.5-inch hypodermic needle. Both acupoints belong to the traditional acupuncture points of bovine and equine systems. Most animals showed heat within 14 days after aquapuncture and were inseminated artificially. They reported that the pregnancy rate after the treatment was 14/18 (77.7%) and 12/18 (66.6%) based on progesterone concentration and rectal palpation respectively, and suggesting acupuncture as a simple and effective method to treat repeat breeders in dairy herds.

11. Reproductive management improvement

Therapeutic management are being used recently for fixed-timed artificial insemination (TAI), without heat detection. These protocols help to treat the cows with silent heats or ovulation problems and all animals are inseminated at a predetermined time. For cows, fixed-timed AI can produce pregnancy rates similar to those of protocols that require 5 to 7 days of heat detection. It is observed that in heifers, pregnancy rates from current TAI protocols tend to be 5 to 10 percent lower than using heat detection alone. The times scheduled for fixed-time AI should be considered as the approximate average time of insemination. This should be based on the number of females to inseminate, labor, and facilities. For these controlled breeding programmes some synthetic hormones are used to control the reproductive cycle of the cow. The following hormones are used in different ways during different programmes.

GnRH (Gonadatrophin Releasing Hormone): This hormone acts on the pituitary gland to stimulate release of FSH and LH. It causes ovulation from the dominant follicle leading to the formation of a corpus luteum which may be available for luteolysis using prostaglandin. It also stimulates the further follicular development through 'new wave emergence' and ovulation takes place from the mature follicles at which the oocyte (egg) is released and optimises the timing of insemination.

Prostaglandin (PG): It acts on the corpus luteum causing it to regress. The corpus luteum produces progesterone and so its destruction causes a sudden drop in the level of progesterone; which removes the inhibition of follicle development and allows a new dominant follicle to mature ready for ovulation in 2-5 days. If there is no CL present then the PG will have no effect.

CIDR or PRID (Intra vaginal Progesterone Releasing Devices): These vaginal implants supply progesterone to the female and so influence the feedback mechanisms of the hypothalamo-pituitary-gonadal axis which inhibits follicle development and ovulation.

hCG (Human Chorionic Gonadatrophin): It has LH-like action to promote ovulation and luteinisation (formation of the CL).

eCG (Equine Chorionic Gonadatrophin): Also known as PMSG (Pregnant Mare Serum Gonadotrophin). It has FSH-like action which stimulates the follicle for recruitment, growth and maturation.

The following methods of oestrus synchronisation with fixed-timed artificial insemination are available, some may carry benefits and some may have draw backs.

Synchronization of oestrus using $PGF_2\alpha$ can improve reproductive efficiency of the animal. In this protocol two prostaglandin injections administered 10-12 days apart, the first PG should cause luteolysis of the corpus luteum present in any cattle beyond day 8 in the ovarian cycle. Cattle will then be returned to the start of the cycle and as such 10-12 days later should have a functioning CL and be receptive to prostaglandin. Many studies have shown that the use of $PGF_2\alpha$ can reduce the interval between detected oestrous cycles and improve estrus detection efficiency. But sometimes $PGF_2\alpha$ does not effectively regress corpora lutea from days 1 to 6 after oestrus; therefore, two injections of $PGF_2\alpha$, administered 11 days apart, are required to effectively synchronize oestrus in dairy heifers. In addition, $PGF_2\alpha$ will not induce estrus in prepubertal heifers because they are lack of corpus luteum. Synchronization of estrus with $PGF_2\alpha$ has been successful if heifers are bred at a detected oestrus (Larson and Ball, 1992), because oestrus detection rates increase and management of AI is more efficient compared with daily oestrus detection. However, oestrus is not precisely synchronized with $PGF_2\alpha$ in dairy heifers because this treatment only regulates the life span of the corpus luteum and it does not worked on growing of follicles. Thus, heifers with functional corpora lutea will exhibit heat from one to six days after treatment with $PGF_2\alpha$. The limitations of this programme are that it results in a relatively wide deviation in time of ovulation from one cow to another and as such double A.I. is recommended at 72 and 96 hours following the second PG. Alternatively the cow can be served once at 84 hours although this can be associated with lower conception rates. The regime is not appropriate if a cow is not cycling normally.

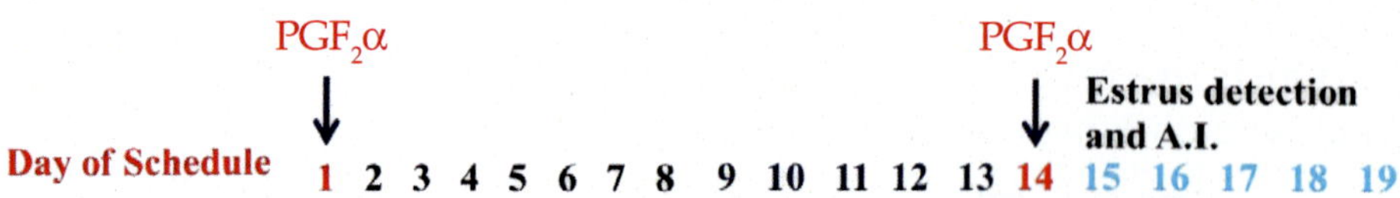

Figure 14. Two doses of prostaglandin injections protocol

Ovsynch was originally developed in the USA and has been used successfully for many years primarily in dairy cattle (Pursley *et al.*, 1995). It represents the blueprint upon which most of the other programs are built. Ovsynch is a protocol based on the administration of GnRH, $PGF_2\alpha$ and GnRH to schedule the insemination time. The first GnRH injection causes ovulation of any dominant follicles leading to CL formation. The PG at 7 days then causes regression of this CL allowing a new dominant follicle to mature before the second GnRH injection 56 hours later causes ovulation ready for fixed time AI. Ambhore *et al.* (2016) reported that by using Ovsynch protocol 91.66% cows exhibited induced oestrus and the fertility rate was 66.67%. By using Ovsynch, dairy producers need not to worry for oestrus detection for timing of AI. The respective cows receive a fixed-time AI in relation to a synchronized ovulation which results in conception rates similar to that of cows receiving AI to a detected oestrus (Pursley *et al.*, 1997a). This fixed-time AI is beneficial to dairy producers who cannot manage oestrus detection adequately and can dramatically improve reproductive efficiency of lactating cows in herds with inadequate AI service rates (Pursley *et al.*, 1997a). But, the dairy heifers respond weakly to Ovsynch and fixed-time AI, exhibiting conception rates 20% to 40% lower than heifers receiving AI to a standing estrus (Pursley *et al.*, 1997b). Therefore, use of Ovsynch and fixed-time AI in dairy heifers is not recommended.

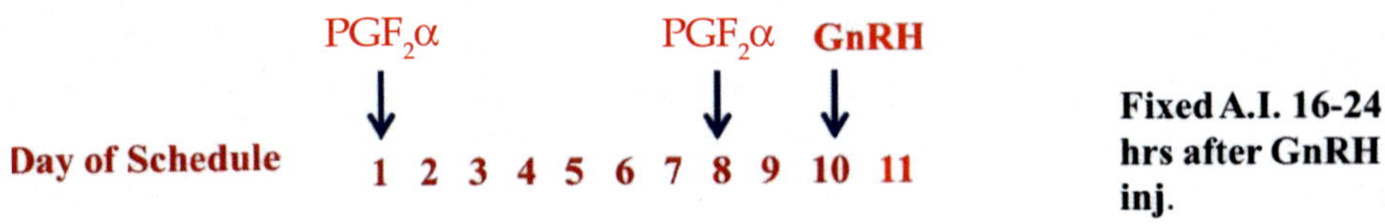

Figure. 15. Ovsynch protocol

Select-synch uses the same protocol as Ovsynch but only cows that are actually observed in oestrus are served. This programme may improve conception rates. However, cows that have ovulated may not be served with a consequent reduction in submission rates, as they may not exhibit oestrogen driven behavioural signs of heat.

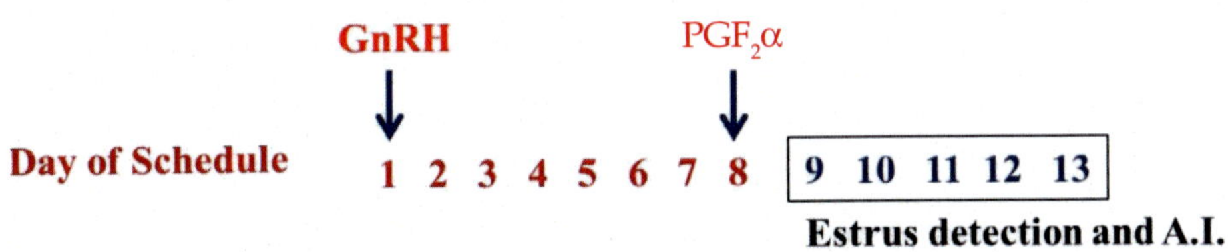

Figure. 16. Select Synch protocol

Co-Synch uses a similar protocol to Ovsynch with the exception that the second injection of GnRH is postponed until 72hours after PG and given at the same time as the cow is served. The benefit of this with regard to beef cattle is that it reduces the number of times that the cattle require handling, thus reducing stress for the cattle as well as reducing labour input.

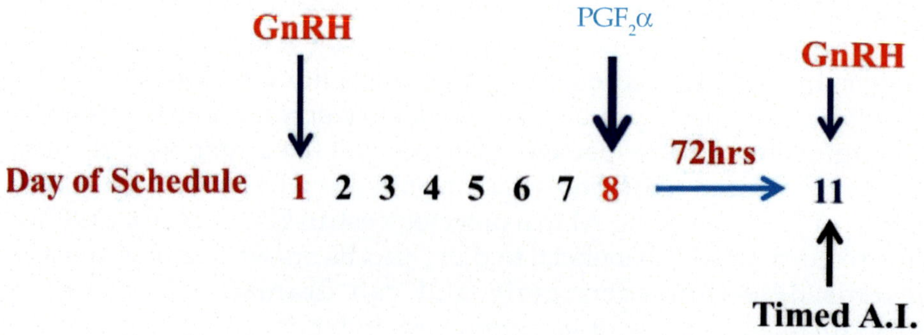

Figure 17. Co-Synch protocol

CIDR-synch uses a CIDR to supplement the levels of natural progesterone produced by the corpus luteum. The CIDR is inserted on day one at the same time as the initial GnRH injection and is left in place for up to 12 days and preceded 24 or preferably 48 hours before withdrawal with an injection of PG. Progesterone supplementation for longer than 12 days may lead to reduced oocyte viability as a consequence of prolonged follicular dominance.

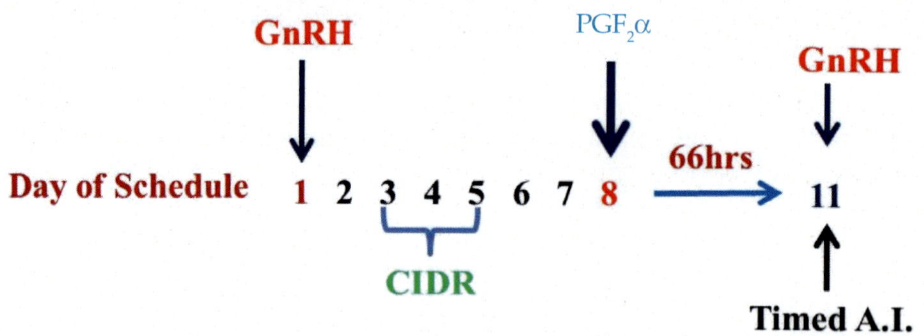

Figure 18. Co-Synch + CIDR protocol

Modified Ovsynch/CIDR-synch uses eCG instead of the first GnRH injection, with FSH action for stimulation of follicular growth and if used in conjunction with intra vaginal progesterone has application in both growing beef heifers and suckle cows synchronised relatively soon post-calving in poor body condition, that calve later in the calving season. A further modification to the programme uses hCG to promote luteinisation and formation of accessory CL to increase progesterone levels post-insemination and reduce embryonic death.

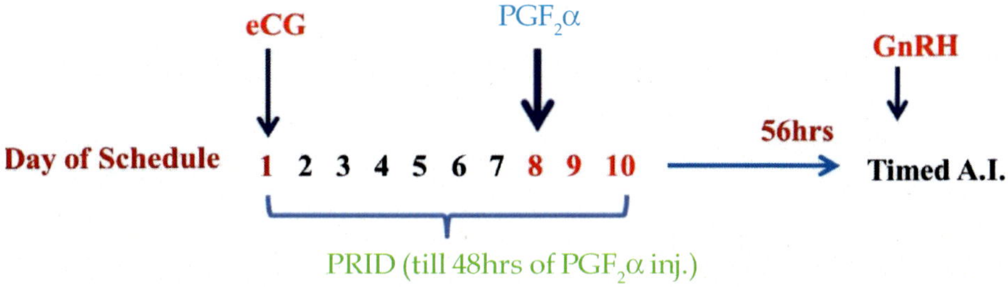

Figure 19. Modified Ovsynch/CIDR-Synch protocol

Triple-synch is a system devised by the Scottish Agricultural College (SAC) which aims is to reduce the need for sweeper bulls by synchronising returns to oestrus by cows that have failed to conceive. Allowing second and third rounds of AI as well as recruiting any late cavers into subsequent rounds of AI. The advantage of this programme is that it gives three opportunities of cows to be served with fixed time AI without the need for a sweeper bull. Disadvantages include labour input and cost. Care must be taken to ensure CIDRs are thoroughly cleaned, disinfected and appropriately stored prior to re-insertion and the modification to a lower progesterone dose in CIDR since first devised may require fresh CIDR inserts at each stage of the programme.

These all protocols help to treat the repeat breeder cows of various etiology and all animals are inseminated at a predetermined time. By using these protocols, dairy producers need not to worry for oestrus detection and also timing of AI. The respective cows receive a fixed-time AI in relation to a synchronized ovulation which results in better conception rates. Various researchers used various methods and off course the success rate is also varied. Ambhore *et al.* (2016) reported that PRID plus Ovsynch protocol with fixed time AI was beneficial than Ovsynch or PRID plus $PGF_2\alpha$ protocol with fertility rate of 75%, 66.67% and 50% respectively. Vijayarajan *et al.* (2016) used Ovsynch plus CIDR protocol with fixed time AI in management of repeat breeding crossbred Jersey cows and they have found that the pregnancy rate in Ovsynch and Ovsynch plus CIDR protocol was 54.54 and 72.72 per cent respectively in comparison to control *i.e.* 27.27 per cent. Rajkumar and Durairajan (2016) reported that the Co- synch method of synchronization with fixed time AI could be effectively used to improve conception rate in repeat breeding cows with 60.00% conception in treated group and 30.00% in control group.

12. Alternative medicinal therapy

As we know, fecundity is one of the key determinants in the life time performance of the dairy animals and reproductive disorders adversely affect the reproductive efficiency of the animal. These disorders may be congenital or acquired. The management options available for the treatment of reproductive disorders include the use of drugs and a variety of surgical procedures. As we have seen in village condition sometimes the poor farmers cannot bear the cost of treatment and even in certain places the suitable drugs are also not available. Moreover due to unavailability or lack of accessibility to veterinary services in the rural areas the farmers had to depend upon the traditional practices for treating their animals. In that case the traditional knowledge of local healers who possess knowledge and experience in traditional systems of treatment become more effective. Many medicinal plants have been claimed to be effective in modulating reproduction. The indigenous traditional knowledge (ITK) of local village communities on medicinal plants helps in curing various reproductive disorders that adversely affect the reproductive efficiency of the livestock. Many medicinal plants have been claimed to be effective in modulating reproduction but the systematic scientific evidence regarding their mechanism of action, dosage or clinical efficacy is lacking. Incorporation of cheap, efficacious and scientifically proven indigenous plant based medicines is the need of the hour along with establishment of their safety needs. The author surveyed the Kamrup district of Assam regarding use of traditional herbal medicines for reproductive disorders of livestock and he found that during acyclicity or irregular in cyclicity of the dairy animals, the farmers used some herbal preparation and gave it along with daily ration to their animals such as

1. About 500 gm cooked Masoor (*Lens culinaris* subsp. *culinaris* syn. *Lens esculenta*) is fed to cattle for 15 days.
2. The green leaves of *Phyllanthus niruri* locally known as Tetali fed to the animals for one week.
3. The fruit of *Mimusops elongi* locally known as Bakul fed to the animals for one week.

In conditions when sufficient nutrients, particularly energy source are not available to the lactating cows, they lost their body condition and as a result there is decrease in milk production and reproductive activity become compromised. In case of pregnant cows the end result is under weight calves and open period postpartum is prolonged. Fertility of the cows declines when they are allowed for breeding in poor condition and ultimately develop repeat breeding. There are various causes of repeat breeding. Out of that nutrition and stress are the major causes. Some of the remedial measures practiced by the farmers which have been documented by Talukdar *et al.* (2015), as mention below:

1. *Citrus aurantifolia* locally known as Kaji nemu is grinded at first and then fed to the animal along with Kala nimakh (black salt) for a month.
2. The green leaves and bark of *Saccharum officinarum* L. locally known as Kuhiyar pat is fed to the animal for one week.
3. A leaf of Pat-kunwar (*Aloe barbadensis* Wall.) is tied externally on the navel portion of the animal.

In certain region of the country, the practitioner also uses some homeopathic medicines which have been recommended also for the management of reproductive disorders. Out of these the Sepia, Calcaria phos, Pulsatila, Alertis ferti, Iodum, Heper sulph, Silica and Oophorinum are used in various doses to treat the metritis, repeat breeding cases in livestock.

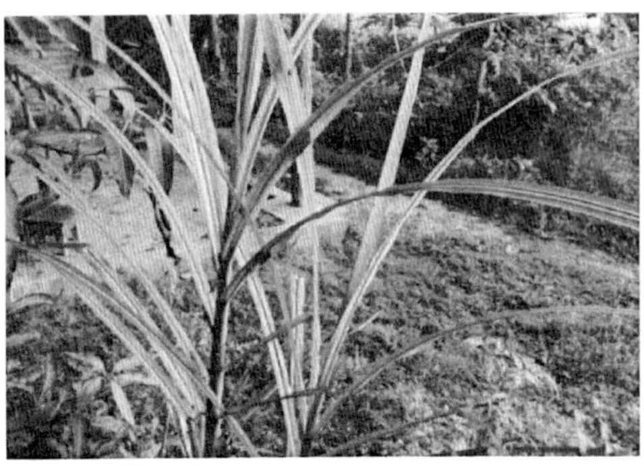

Saccharum officinarum
(Sugar cane)

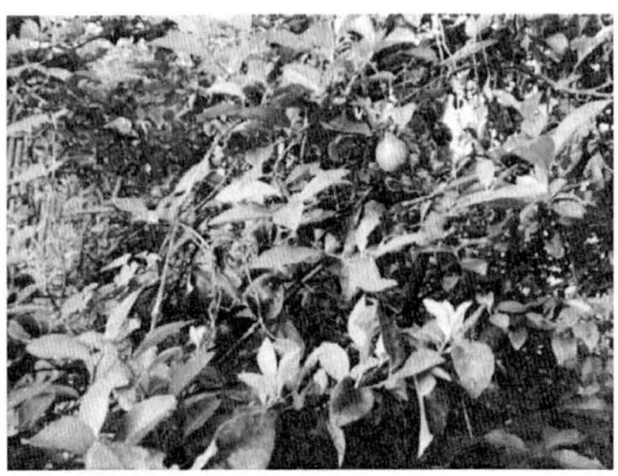

Citrus aurantifolia
(Lemon)

Figure 20. Commonly use herbs for reproductive problems in Cattle by the farmers

Summary

After therapeutic management of repeat breeding problem it is necessary to continually monitor the conditions in the herd to insure that the problem is not recurring. Thus, the records must be kept up-to-date to allow for ongoing evaluation of the herd's reproductive performance.

Inadequate oestrus detection is the most frequent cause of repeat breeding. Detection of estrus is of great important especially in a herd being bred by A.I. It is also essential to improve all aspects related to heat detection, since it has been established that oestrus detection mistakes reduces the reproductive capacity of the dairy cows. Therefore, it could be interesting to implement different methods for oestrus detection as Kamar or Bovine Heat-beacon devices, chin-ball marker, tail chalking, milk progesterone tests, androgenised animals and pedometers as well as the cows should be watched closely for estrum at least twice daily at morning and evening. Heat expectancy chart or the regular examinations of the genital tract of open cows by the veterinarian are very helpful to predict the time of estrus. If it is not possible then we can go for fixed timed artificial insemination by using some exogenous hormonal compound. Whatever the protocol followed, the cows should be bred at the proper time of each oestrus period with highly fertile bull or bull semen to achieve the best and early conception rates.

All the animals in the herd should be examined at each regular monthly, or more frequently specially those cows which is repeated. The herdsman should be in touch with the local veterinarian for determination of pregnancy if breeding has taken place 35 or more days ago. The animals that fail to conceive due to any pathological condition such as metritis, adhesion of the oviduct, cystic ovaries and other lesions or diseases, including anoestrus may be treated or culled.

The cleanliness at the time of calving is very important in respect to prevent postpartum uterine infections and delayed conception. Otherwise the economy of the farm goes down. It is very important that the diseased animal should be separated from the healthy one as early. In this cases we can use various advanced diagnostic tools and appliances for easy and early diagnosis so that we can maintain a disease free herd as well as minimize the incidence of repeat breeding which may be infected origin. For that a strict monitoring should also be needed and proper and regular vaccination should also be done.

Highly fertile, active bulls with a strong sex drive and free of infectious venereal diseases should be used as sire. If A.I. is employed the fertility record of the bull should be noted. The semen should be stored, handled, thawed and inseminated in a manner to maintain and promote the high fertility of the spermatozoa.

The herdsman who is in daily close continuous contact with the herd is the most important person for determining the various reproductive problems associated with the dairy herds. So, frequent observation is required. He is the person who is properly educated and motivated for successful of the dairy industry.

The optimum herd reproductive parameters of the farm should be:

1.	Age at first estrus/puberty	12-18 months
2.	Age at first breeding	18-24 months
3.	Age at first calving	30-36 months
4.	Days open	Less than 110 days
5.	Calving interval	12-13 months
6.	Calving to first observed estrus	<45 days
7.	First service conception rate	>50%
8.	Service per conception	Less than 1.7
9.	Calving to conception	<90 days
10.	Abortions	<4%
11.	Retained placenta incidence	<8%
12.	Uterine infection	<10%
13.	Cystic ovarian disease incidence	<10%
14.	Repeat breeding	<15%

❑❑❑

Appendix

A. Reproductive characteristics of Domestic Animals

Animal	Onset of Puberty	Length of Oestrous Cycle	Length of Estrum	Time of ovulation	Optimum time for service	Fertile life of sperm in female tract	Fertile life of ovum
Cow	1-2 $^1/_2$ years	18-24 days (21days)	12-24hrs (18 hrs)	10-12 hrs after end of oestrus	mid to end of oestrus (12 hr after the onset of heat)	30-48 hrs	20-24 hrs
She buffalo	2 $^1/_2$ years	21 days	12-30 hrs (20 hrs)	15-18 hrs after end of oestrus	mid to end of oestrus (12 hr after the onset of heat)	30-48 hrs	12-24 hrs
Mare	18-24 months (18 months)	19-23 days (21 days)	4- 7days	1-2 days before end of oestrus	2nd or 3rd day of oestrus	72- 120 hrs (3-5 days)	6-8 hrs
Ewe	6-9 months	14-20 days (17 days)	24-36 hrs	24-27 hrs after onset of heat	18-24 hrs after the onset of oestrus	30-48 hrs	16-24 hrs
Goat	6- 8 months (Pygmy goats 3 months)	18-24 days (21 days)	24-48 hrs	30-36 hrs after onset of heat	24-36hrs after the onset of oestrus	24- 48 hrs	12-24 hrs
Sow	5-8 months	18-24 days (21 days)	2-3 days	35-45 hrs after onset of heat	12-30 hrs after the onset of heat	24-72 hrs	8-10 hrs
Bitch	6-12 months	Monoestrus	4-13 days (9 days)	24-72 hrs after LH surge	2-3 days after the onset of true oestrus	4-7 days	4-7 days

Source: Hafez E.S.E., 1993. Reproduction in Farm Animals, 6th Edn., Lea and Febiger, Philadelphia.

B. Average gestation period in different animals

Animal	Gestation periods (Days)
Cow	270-285
Buffalo	305-315
Sheep	145-155
Goat	145-152
Sow	114
Mare	335-345
Bitch	62-64
Camel	333-430
Elephant	615-650
Rhinoceros	530-548

Source: Hafez E.S.E., 1993. Reproduction in Farm Animals, 6th Edn., Lea and Febiger, Philadelphia.

C. Average duration of reproductive life in domestic animals

Animal	Reproductive life
Dairy Cow	8-10 years
Buffalo	12 years
Sheep	6-10 years
Goat	15-18 years
Sow	6-8 years
Mare	18-22 years
Bitch	8-12 years

Source: Hafez E.S.E., 1993. Reproduction in Farm Animals, 6th Edn., Lea and Febiger, Philadelphia.

D. Normal haematological parameters in dairy cattle

Parameters	Normal range
Red blood cells (RBC)	5- 10 × 10^6 cells/µl
Haemoglobin (Hb)	08- 15 g/dl
Haematocrit (PCV)	24- 46 %
White blood cells (WBC)	4-12 × 10^3 cells/µl
Neutrophils (band)	0- 2 %
Neutrophils (segmented)	15- 45 %
Lymphocytes	45- 75 %
Monocytes	2- 7 %
Eosinophils	2- 20 %
Basophils	0- 2 %
Platelets	01- 08 × 10^5 /µl

Source: Merck's Veterinary Manual

E. Normal blood biochemical values for cattle

Parameters	Normal range
Random glucose (mg/dL)	40 - 100
Total protein (gm/dL)	6.7 - 7.5
Albumin (gm/dL)	2.5 - 3.8
Globulin (gm/dL)	3 - 3.5
ALT (u/L)	6.9 - 35
AST (u/L)	60 - 125
ALP (u/L)	18 - 153
SDH (u/L)	4.3 - 15.3
Total Bilirubin (mg/dL)	0 - 1.6
Direct Bilirubin(mg/dL)	0.04 - 0.44
BUN (mg/dL)	10 - 25
Creatinine (u/L)	0.5 - 2.2
Cholesterol (mg/dL)	62 - 193
Amylase (u/L)	41 - 98
CPK (u/L)	0 - 350
LDH (u/L)	309 - 938

Source: Merck's Veterinary Manual

F. Hormones used in Animal Reproduction

Hormone	Indication, dose and route	Presentation
I. Gonadotropin Releasing Hormone (GnRH)		
Endogenous GnRH – • Decapeptide • Secreted by the hypothalamus • Stimulates FSH & LH release from the anterior pituitary gland Buserelin, Fertirelin and Gonadorelin are the synthetic analogues of GnRH	**Buserelin** (GnRH Analouge) • Anestrum (Cattle) - 20 µg, IV or IM. Repeat after 8-22 days if required. • Delayed ovulation (Cattle) -10 µg, IV or IM. • Improvement of conception rate (Cattle) 5 - 10 µg, IV or IM. Before or at the time of insemination. • Cystic ovaries with or without symptom of nymphomania (Cattle) - 20 µg, IV or IM. Repeat after 8-14 days if required.	• **Receptal** (MSD) Contains Buserelin 4µg/ml. Vials of 2.5 ml and 10 ml. • **Gynarich** (Intas) Contains Buserelin Acetate 4µg/ml. Vials of 2.5 ml and 5 ml. • **Pregulate** (Virbac) Each ml contains Buserelin IP - 0.004mg, Benzyl Alcohol IP (as preservative) - 10mg. Vials of 5 ml. • **Gynofertin** (Bovian) Each ml contains Buserelin Acetate 4.2µg. Vials of 2.5 ml.

		• **Ovulanta Inj.** (Vet Mankind) Each ml contains Buserelin Acetate 4µg. Vials of 2.5 & 5 ml.
II. Luteinizing hormone (LH) • Glycoprotein. • Secreted by the anterior pituitary gland in both male and females. • Human Chorionic Gonadotropin (hCG) having LH like activity which is widely used.	**In female** (Cattle): Delayed ovulation, Prolonged estrusAnovulation = 1500 -3000IU at the time of insemination, IV or IM. Follicular cyst = 3000 IUI/ M or IV. **In male:** Deficient libido1500 IU IM twice weekly for 4- 6 weeks.	• **Chorulon** (MSD) Injection: Powder for reconstitution. Contains Chorionic gonadotropin. 1500 IU/vial • **LH 1500** (Paines & Byrne) Injection: Powder for reconstitution. Contains Chorionic gonadotropin. 1500 IU/vial
III. Follicle Stimulating homone (FSH) • Glycoproteins • Pregnant Mare Serum Gonadotropin (PMSG) or Equine ChorionicGonadotropin (eCG) having predominantly FSH like activity and little LH like activity.	• Anestrous (cattle): 500 – 1000 IU, IM. • Induction of superovulation: 1500- 3000 IU, IM, between day 8- 13 of the cycle, followed by PGF2α after 48 hrs.	• **Folligon** (MSD) Injection: Powder for reconstitution. Serum gonadotropin. 1000 IU/vial. • **Follitropin – V** (Bioniche, Canada) – contains FSH equivalent to 400 mg NIH / vial. • **Trophovet** (Indian Immunologicals) Contains PMSG 1000 IU/Vial
IV. Prostaglandins • Causes functional and morphological regression of the CL. • Natural prostaglandins and synthetic analogues are available	• Induction of ovulation • Synchronization of estrus • Termination of pregnancy • Induction of parturition • Persistent CL • Mummified fetus • Pyometra • Luteal cyst • Embryo transfer Natural – 25 mg IM Synthetic analouge –0.5 mg (2 ml) IM (Cattle)	• **Natural** (Novartis) Lutalyse Dinoprost-tromethamine Contains 5 mg/ml Vials of 10ml, 30ml • **Dinofertin injection** (Alved) Contains 5mg/ml. Vials of 5 ml. • **Synthetic Estrumate** (Coopers Pitman – Moore) Cloprostenol (as sodium salt) Contains 250µg/ml, Vials of 2ml, 10ml and 20ml. • **Cyclix/ Estrumate** (MSD) contains Cloprostenol 0.263 mg /ml. Vials of 2ml and 20ml.

		• **Synchromate** (Prima Vet care) contains Cloprostenol - 263µg/ ml. Vial of 4ml. • **Vetmate** (Virbac) Contains Cloprostenol 263 µg/ml. Vial of 2 ml. • **Pragma** (Intas)Contains Cloprostenol 250 µg/ ml.Vial of 2 ml. • **Clostenol Injection** (Zydus AH) contains Cloprostenol 263 µg/ml. Vial of 2 ml. • **Pregova** (Virbac) contains Cloprostenol 263 µg/ml. Vial of 2 ml. • **Gynostart** (Bovian) contains Cloprostenol 263 µg/ml. Vial of2 ml.
V. Progesterone • Steroids • Maintain pregnancy • Inhibit oestrus and ovulation	• To improve fertility and conception rate. 250 to 500 mg of depot preparation IM on the 4th day of AI. • To prevent threatened abortions 500 mg of depot preparation, IM. Repeat 4-5 times at every 10-15 days interval until 7 months. • Intravaginal device CIDR, PRID, Ear Implant-Syncro -Mate-B. • Estrus induction/Synchro-nization/Anestrum/ Cystic ovaries.	• **Eazi Breed CIDR** Intravaginal device 1.38 gm progesterone 7–12 days with/without PG at the time of removal. • **PRID** (Sanofi) Intravaginal device Progestrone 1.55g. + Oestradiol benzoate 10 mg. Removed after 12 days followed by AI. • **Syncro-Mate-B.** (Sanofi) contains 6mg of norgestomet for the ear implant with injection of 5mg of estradiol valerate and 3mg of norgestomet for IM use. (a single 2ml dose). Implant removed after 9 days followed by AI. • **Crestar** (MSD) Crestar implant contains 3 mg of progestagen Norgestomet. Crestar inj. 2ml Contains ml 3 mg Norgestomet and 5 mg oestradiol valerate.

		• **TRIU-B** (Virbac) Each device comprises of 3 medicated rings (green colour) containing Progesterone IP 186 mg each and one additional ring (pink colour) with Progesterone IP 400 mg. Place the device inside the applicator tube. Insert the applicator tube into vagina. Expel the device in vagina and the applicator. Presentation : 10 units/ carton **Hydroxy progesterone caproate:** • **Duraprogen injection** (Virbac) 250 /mg/ml. 2ml amp. (depot) • **Hyprogen** (Vets farma) 250/ mg/ml. 2ml, 3ml amp. • **Proluton Depot** (German Remedies) 250 mg/ml. 2ml amp. • **P-Depot Injection** (Zydus AH) 250mg/ml 2ml and 3ml amp.
VI. Oxytocin • Peptide hormone • Milk letting down • Smooth muscle contraction • Uterus • Myoepithelial cells of the mammary gland	• Large Animals Milk letdown (5 - 10 Units) Retained Placenta (30 - 50 Units. Primary Uterine interia (30 - 50 Units. • Small Animals - Uterine inertia 10 units(small doses repeatedly)	• **Pitocin** (Parke -Davis) 5 IU / 0.5ml/ amp • Syntocinon (Novartis) 5 IU / ml., 1 ml amp
VII. Clomiphene Citrate • Non - steroidal compound • Remarkable structural similarity to Estradiol (E2) and • Antiestrogenic by competing with estrogens • Binds to the E2 receptors in the hypothalamus to create	Induction of Ovulation • Anestrus 300 mg tab/ orally for 3 - 5 days (after administration of 1% Copper Sulphate Solution) • Repeat Breeding 300 mg 3 - 5 days (after administration of 1% Copper Sulphate Solution)	• **Clofert** (Sigma labs) Tab 25 mg, 50 mg, 100 mg. Clofert Vet - 300 mg • **Clone** (Chemech) Tab. 25mg, 50mg, 100mg, 150mg • **Fertivet** (Cipla) Tab. 300 mg. Cisclompiphene citrate - 180mg, Transclomiphene citrate 120 mg.

a state of hypoestrogenicity, hereby causing an enhanced Gonadotropin releasing hormone (GnRH) release followed by an increased secretion of gonadotropins which induces ovulation.		• **Fertomid** (Cipla) Tab 25mg, 50 mg • **Siphene** (serum Institute) Tab 500 mg, 100 mg • **Ovulanta-Kit** (Vet Mankind) Each kit contains one tablet of Clomifene citrate 300mg + two tablet of Copper sulphate pentahydrate 750mg.
VIII. Oestradiol analogue • Natural steroidal oestrogens include oestradiols, oestrone and oestriols. They have low oral activity and so simple esters of steroidal oestrogens such as benzoates or valerates are used in therapeutics as they release parent molecule on hydrolysis. • Induces oestrus, parturition.	• Treatment of reproductive disorders like anoestrus & sub-oestrus • Synchronisation of oestrus • To stimulate uterine expulsion of retained placenta and mummified foetus.	• **Pregheat** (Virbac) Each ml contains Oestradiol Benzoate IP - 1 mg, Benzyl Alcohol IP (as preservative) - 0.1 ml. Arachis Oil IP - q.s. **Cattle:** 2 ml Pregheat equivalent to 2 mg Oestradiol Benzoate per animal intramuscularly. Vial of 5ml. • **Heatreg injection** (Novitech) Contains Diethylstilbestrol 10 mg/ mlFor induction oestrus, Cattle , Buffalo= 1.5 ml on day 1 and 1.5 ml after 3 days, IM.For induction of parturition, pyometra and retention of placenta Cattle , Buffalo= 3 ml IM Vial of 3 ml

N.B. Compiled from the various sources.

G. Certain drugs used in Animal Reproduction specially in reproductive disorder in Cattle

Sl. No.	Category	Product name	Ingredient	Indication	Present-ation	Manufac-turer
1	Intrauterine (Suspension)	CFlox-TZ IU	Ciprofloxacin hydrochloride 125 mg + Tinidazole 150 mg/ 5ml	Repeat breeding of infective origin, metritis, pyometra, retention of placenta, other reproductive tract infections. **Dose:** 30-60 ml by intra-uterine route. Repeat twice at an interval of 24 hours.	60ml bottles	Neovet – Intas Pharmace-utical
2	Intrauterine (Suspension)	Lenovo AP	Levofloxacin 100mg + Ornidazole 200mg + Vitamin E 25mg/5ml	Repeat breeding of infective origin, metritis, pyometra, retention of placenta, other reproductive tract infections. **Dose:** 30-60 ml by intra-uterine route. Repeat twice at an interval of 24 hours.	30 and 60 ml bottles	Neovet – Intas Pharmace-utical
3	Intrauterine (Suspension)	Metric-are IU	Povidone Iodine IP: 5% w/v Metroni-dazole IP: 1% w/v	Repeat breeding of infective origin, metritis, pyometra, retention of placenta, other reproductive tract infections and in uterine prolapse as topical application. **Dose:** 30-60 ml by intra-uterine route. Repeat twice at an interval of 24 hours.	30 ml & 100 ml bottles	Zydus AH
4	Intrauterine (Suspension)	Wokad-ine IU	Povidone Iodine 5% w/v, Metronidazole 1% w/v	Repeat breeding of infective origin, metritis, pyometra, retention of placenta and other reproductive tract infections. **Dose:** Cattle=30-60 ml by intra-uterine route.	60 ml bottle	Vetoquinol
5	Intrauterine (Bolus)	Furex	Nitrofurazone 60gm+Urea 6gm	Metritis, pyometra, cervicitis, vaginitis, retention of placenta **Dose**: Cattle=2-4 boli	Bolus 4's	Vetsfarma
6	Intrauterine (Bolus)	Furex-M	Nitrofurazone 60 gm+Urea	Metritis, pyometra, cervicitis, vaginitis,	Bolus 4's	Vetsfarma

			5 gm+Metronidazole 1gm	retention of placenta **Dose**: Cattle=2-4 boli		
7	Ecbolic	Nexbolic injection	Methylergometrine Maleate 1 mg/ml	Postpartum atony, haemorrhage and subinvolution of uterus. Helps in expulsion of placenta and facilitates lochial discharge thus minimize the risk of postpartum metritis. **Dose:** Cow & Mare = 2-5 mg/ animal by IV or IM	5 ml vial	Neovet – Intas Pharmaceutical
8	Ecbolic	Ergometrin Injection	Each ml contains: Methyl Ergometrine Maleate IP : 1 mg	Retained placenta, post-partum metritis or pyometra, for expulsion of lochial discharge. **Dose:** Cow & Mare = 2-5 mg/animal by IV or IM route	5 ml vial	Zydus AH
9	Anti cholinergic	Epidosin injection	Valethmate 10 mg/ ml	Hard cervix and inadequate cervical dilatation during parturition, to prevent cervical and vaginal tear. **Dose:** Cattle, Mare = 40- 50mg, IM	10 ml and 30 ml	TTK
10	Uterine tonic and cleansing agent	Exaper Bolus and Liquid*		Retained placenta, delayed involution of uterus. **Dose:** Cattle, Mare= 2-4 boli BID, 100ml followed by 50ml BID in case of liquid preparation.	Bolus 4's, 500ml bottle	Ayurvet
11	Uterine tonic and cleansing agent	Involone Bolus and Liquid*		Retained placenta, delayed involution of uterus. **Dose:** Cattle, Mare = 1 bolus BID, 200ml followed by 100ml in case of liquid preparation.	Bolus 6's, 500ml, 1 liter and 5 liter.	Natural Remedies
12	Uterine tonic and cleansing agent	Replanta powder*		Retained placenta, delayed involution of uterus. **Dose:** Cattle, Buffalo = 100gm initial dose followed by 50-60 gm QID	100gm, 500gm powder	Indian Herbs
13	Oestrus inducer	Bucofert*		Infertility associated with ovarian	Bolus 6's	Natural Remedies

			dysfunctions like anoestrus, silent heat, delayed puberty and infective conditions. **Dose:** Cow= 2 boli/day for 3 days. Repeat on 11th, 12th & 13th day in case of no oestrus signs.		
14	Oestrus inducer	Janova*	Infertility associated with ovarian dysfunctions like anoestrus, silent heat, delayed puberty and infective conditions. **Dose:** Cow= 3 cap/day for 2 days. Repeat after 10 days in case of absence of oestrus.	Capsule 6's	Ayurvet
15	Oestrus inducer	Prajana HS*	Infertility associated with ovarian dysfunctions like anoestrus, silent heat, and delayed puberty. **Dose:** Cow= 3 cap/day for 2 days. Repeat after 10 days in case of absence of oestrus.	Capsule 6's	Indian Herbs
16	Oestrus inducer	Sajani*	Infertility associated with ovarian dysfunctions like anoestrus, silent heat, and delayed puberty. **Dose:** Cow= 3 cap/day for 2 days. Repeat after 10 days in case of absence of oestrus.	Capsule 6's	Zydus AH
17	Oestrus inducer	Uterotone capsule*	Infertility associated with ovarian dysfunctions like anoestrus, silent heat, delayed puberty . **Dose:** Cow= 4 cap/day for 4 days. Repeat after 10 days if necessary.	Capsule 8's	Cattle remedies

N.B. Compiled from the various sources.

**For composition visit company web site.*

❑❑❑

References

A. K. Sarkar. (2006). Therapeutic management of anoestrus cows with diluted Lugol's iodine and massage on reproductive organs. *J. Anim. Vet. Sci.,* **1**(1): 30-32.

Ahmad, N.; S. W. Beam; W. R. Butler; D. R. Deaver; R. T. Duby; E. Elder; J. E. Fortune; L. C. Griel; L. S. Jones; R. A. Milvae; L. Pate; I. Revah; D. T. Scheriber; D. H. Townson; P. C. W. Tasnag and E. K. Inskeep. (1996). Relationships of fertility to patterns of ovarian follicular development and associated hormonal profiles in dairy cows and heifers. *J. Anim. Sci.* **74**: 1943-1952.

Ahmed, W. M.; El-khadrawy, H. H.; Emtenan, M.; Ali, A. H. and Shalaby, S. A. (2010). Clinical perspective of repeat breeding syndrome in buffaloes. *J. Anim. Sci.,* **6**: 11.

Albihn, A. (1991). Standing oestrus, ovarian function and early pregnancy in virgin and repeat breeding heifers. *J Vet. Med.,* **38**: 212-221.

Ali, A.; Abdul- Razek, A. K.; Derar, R.; Abdul- Rheem, H. A. and Shehata, S. H. (2009). Forms of reproductive disorders in cattle and buffaloes in Middle Egypt.*Reprod. Domest. Anim.,* **44**: 580-585.

Ambhore, G.S.; Shelar, R.R.; Pawshe, C.H. and Kapadnis, P.J. (2016). Comparative efficacy of ovysnch, PRID device + PGF2á and PRID + ovysnch based estrus induction protocol on reproductive performance in Dangi cows. *In*: Compendium, XXXII Annual convention of ISSAR, pp.29.

Amiridis, G. S.; Tsiligiamni, T. H.; Dovolou, E.; Rekkas, C.; Vouzaros, D. and Menegatos, I. (2009). Combined administration of gonadotropin- releasing hormone, progesterone and meloxicam is an effective treatment for the repeat- breeder cow. *Theriogenology,* **72**: 542-548.

Awasthi, M. K.; Kavani, F. S.; Siddiquee, G. M.; Dhami, A. J. and Sarvariya, N.P. (2007). Detection of early embryonic mortality through ultrasound scanning in water buffaloes. *Indian J. Anim. Reprod.,* **28**: 26-29.

Baker, D. H. and Ammerman, C. B. (1995). Zinc availability: In : Bioavailability of nutrients for animals. (C.B. Ammerman, D.H. Baker & A.J. Lewis, eds). Academic Press, San Diego, pp. 367-398.

Bartlett, P. C.; Krik, J. H. and Mather, E. C. (1986). Repeated insemination in Michingan Holstein- Friesian cattle: incidence, descriptive epidemiology and estimated economic impact. *Theriogenology,* **26**: 309-322.

Bazer, F.W.; Wu, G.; Johnson, G.A. and Wang, X. (2014). Environmental factors affecting pregnancy: endocrine disrupters, nutrients and metabolic pathways. *Mol. Cell. Endocrinol.,* **398**: 53-68.

Berry, D.P.; Friggens, N.C.; Lucy, M. and Roche, J.R. (2016). Milk Production and Fertility in Cattle. *Annual Review of Animal Biosciences,* **4**: 269-290.

Boland, M.P.; Lonergan, P. and Callaghan, O. (2001). Effect of nutrition on endocrine parameters, ovarian physiology, and oocyte and embryo development. *Theriogenology,* **55**: 1323-1340.

Bulman, D.C. and Lamming G.E. (1978). Milk progesterone levels in relation to conception, repeat breeding and factors influencing acyclity in dairy cows. *J. Reprod. Fert.,* **54**: 447-458.

Butler, S. T. (2014). Nutritional management to optimize fertility of dairy cows in pasture-based systems. *Animal,* **8**(1): 15–26.

Butler, W. R. (1998). Review: effect of protein nutrition on ovarian and uterine physiology in dairy cattle. *J. Dairy Sci.,* **81**: 2533-2539.

Butler, W. R. (2005). Relationships of Dietary Protein and Fertility. *Advances in Dairy Technology,* **17**: 159-168.

Capuco, A.V.; Wood, D.L.; Bright, S.A.; Miller, R.H. and Britman, J. (1990). Regeneration of teat canal keratin in lactating dairy cows. *Journal of dairy science,* **73**: 1051-1057.

Chaffaux, S.; Valon, F. and Martinez, J. (1982). *In:* Evolution de l´image echographique du produit de conception chez la vache. *Bull Acad. Vet.,* **55**: 213-221.

Chagas, L. M.; Bass, J. J. and Blache, D. (2007). Invited review: new perspectives on the roles of nutrition and metabolic priorities in the subfertility of high-producing dairy cows. *Journal of Dairy Science,* **90**(9): 4022–4032.

Chandra,G.; Aggarwal, A.; Singh, A. K.; Kumar, M.; Kushwaha, R.; Singh, A. and Singh, Y. K. (2011). Negative energy balance and reproduction: A review. *Agri. Reviews,* **32**(4): 246-254.

Close, W.H. (1998). The role of organic trace mineral proteinates in pig nutrition. In: Biotechnology in the Feed Industry. Proc. Alltech's 14th Annual Symp. pp. 469-483.

Cromwell, G.L. (1997). In : Handbook of copper compounds and applications. Pp. 177-202.

Daniel, R.C.W. (1983). Motility of the rumen and abomasums during hypocalcemia. *Canadian Journal of Comparative Medicine and Veterinary Science,* **47**: 267-280.

Deka, K. C. (1994). Studies on certain aspect of ovulatory disturbances in repeat breeding crossbred cattle. Ph. D. thesis, Assam Agril. Univ., Guwahati, Assam.

Dhabale, R.B.; Sharma, N. C.; and Sharma, T. (2000). Serum progesterone level in repeat breeding cows. *Indian J. Anim. Reprod.,* **21**(1): 67.

Diskin, M. G.; Mackey, D. R.; Roche, J. F. and Sreenan, J. M. (2003). Effects of nutrition and metabolic status on circulating hormones and ovarian follicle development in cattle. *Animal Reproduction Science,* **78**(3): 345–370.

Do, V.H. and Taylor, R. A.W. (2015). Influence of Maternal Nutritional Factors on Ovarian Folliculogenesis in Cattle. *J. Vet. Sci. Anim. Husb.* **3**(3): 301.

Duchens, M.; Maciel, M.; Gustafsson, H.; Forsberg, M.; Rodriguez-Martinez, H. and Edqvist, L. (1995). Influence of perioestrous suprabasal progesterone levels on cycle length, oestrous behaviour and ovulation in heifers. *Anim. Reprod. Sci.,* **37**: 95-108.

Duffy, P.; Crowe, M.A.; Austin, E.J.; Mihm, M.; Boland, M.P. and Roche, J.F. (2004). The effect of eCG or estradiol at or after norgestomet removal on follicular dynamics, estrus and ovulation in early post-partum beef cows nursing calves. *Theriogenology,* **61**: 725-734.

Dunn, T.G. and Moss, G.E. (1992). Effects of nutrient deficiencies and excesses on reproductive efficiency of livestock. *Journal of Animal Science,* **70**: 1580-1593.

El- Belely, M.S. (1993). Progesterone, estrogen and selected biochemical constituents in plasma and uterine flushings of normal and repeat breeder buffalo cows. *J. Agri. Sci.,* **120**: 241-250.

Elrod, C.C. and Butler, W.R. (1993). Reduction of fertility and alteration of uterine pH in heifers fed excess ruminally degradable protein. *Journal of Animal Science,* **71**: 694-701.

Garcia-Garcia, R. M. (2012). Integrative Control of Energy Balance and Reproduction in Females. *In*: International Scholarly Research Network, ISRN Veterinary Science, Article ID 121389, doi:10.5402/2012/121389.

Goff, J.P. (1999). Dry cow nutrition and metabolic disease in parturient cows. In: Proceeding Western Canadian Dairy Seminar Red Deer. pp. 177-202.

Gunn, P. J.; Lemenager, R. P.; Taylor, E. G. and Bridges, G. A. (2014b). Excess rumen undegradable protein alters parameters of reproductive function in beef cows. *In:* Iowa State Univ. Anim. Industry Report. AS 660, ASL R 2852.

Gunn, P. J.; Lundberg, A.L.; Cushman, R. A.; Freetly, H. C.; Amundson, O. L.; Walker, J. A. and Perry, G. A. (2016). Effect of circulating blood or plasma urea nitrogen concentrations on reproductive efficiency in beef heifers and cows. *In:* Iowa State University animal industry report: AS 662, ASL R3066. Available at: *http://lib.dr.iastate.edu/ans_air/vol662/iss1/27.*

Gupta, J., Dabas, Y.P.S., Lakhchaura, B.D., and Maurya, S.N. (1998). Estradiol- 17 ß and progesterone profile in repeat breeding cattle. *Indian J. Anim. Reprod.,* **19**(2): 126-128.

Gustafsson, H. and Emanuelson, U. (2002). Characterization of the repeat breeding syndrome in Swedish dairy cattle. *Acta Vet. Scand.,***43**: 115-125.

Hammon, D.S.; Holyoak, G.R. and Dhiman, T.R. (2004). Association between blood plasma urea nitrogen levels and reproductive fluid urea nitrogen and ammonia concentrations in early lactation dairy cows. *Anim. Reprod. Sci.,* **59**: 23-30.

Hanafi, E. M.; Ahmed, W.M.; Sherein, I. A. E.; Elkhadrawy, H. H. and Abd El Hameed, A. R. (2008). Effect of clinical endometritis on ovaries activity and oxidative stress status in Egyptian buffalo cows. *Am. Eurasian J. Agric. Environ. Sci.,* **4**: 530-536.

Hansen, P. J. (2016). Influence of Dietary Protein and Amino Acids on Reproduction in Dairy Cows. *WCDS Advances in Dairy Technology,* **28**: 209-216.

Harmon, R.J. (1998). Trace minerals and dairy cattle: importance for udder health. In: Biotechnology in the Feed Industry. Proc Alltech's 14th Annual Symp. Pp. 485-495.

Hemken, R.W.; Harmon, R.J. and Trammell, S. (1998). Selenium for dairy cattle : a role for organic selinium. In: Biotechnology in the Feed Industry. Proc. Alltech's 14th Annual Symp. Pp. 497-503.

Hemler, M.E. and Lands, W.E.M. (1980). Evidence of peroxide-initiated free radical mechanism of prostaglandin biosynthesis. *Journal of Biological chemistry,* **225**: 6253-6261.

Hess, B.W.; Moss, G.E. and Rule, D.C. (2008). A decade of developments in the area of fat supplementation research with beef cattle and sheep. *Journal of Animal Science,* **86**: 188-204.

Hewett, C. D. (1968). A survey of the incidence of the repeat breeder cows in Sweden with referenceto herd size, season, age and milk yield. *British Vet. J.,***124**: 342-352.

Honparkhe, M.; Gandotra, V.K. and Nanda, A.S. (2004). Ultrasonographic measurements in comparison with the rectal palpation and echotexture of reproductive organs of buffaloes (Bubalus bubalis) during different stages of the estrous cycle. *Asian-Aust J Anim Sci.,* **17**: 919-923.

Hosaha, T. and Nakama, S. (2002). Effects of moxibustion for reproductive failure in dairy cattle. *In:* XXII World Buiatrics Congress, Hannover, Germany, pp. 212.

Hwang, Y. and Egerbacher, M. (2001). Anatomy and Classification of Acupoints. In: Veterinary Acupuncture Ancient Art to Modern Medicine, Schoen AM (Ed.), Mosby, pp. 19-25.

Ingraham, R.H.; Kappel, L.C.; Morgan, E.B. and Srikandakumar, A. (1987). Correction of subnormal fertility with copper and magnesium supplementation. *J. Dairy Sci.* **70**: 167-180.

Jackson, P.G.G. and Cockcroft, P.D. (2002). Laboratory Reference Values: Biochemistry. *In:* Clinical Examination of Farm Animals, Blackwell Science Ltd, pp. 303-305.

Joe, A. A.; D. Kathiresan; T.G. Devanathan; R.C. Rajasundaram and J, Rajasekaran. (1998). Blood biochemical profile in normal cyclical and anoestrous cows. *Indian. J. Anim. Sci.,* **68**: 1154-1156.

Jousan, F.D.; Utt, M.D. and Beal, W.E. (2002). Effects of differences in dietary protein on the production and quality of bovine embryos collected from superovulated donors. *Journal of Animal Science,* **8**: 1.

Kaitenbach, C. C. and T. G. Dunn. (1980). Reproduction in farm animals, 4th Edn. Ed. E.S.E. Hafez. Philadelphia and Febiger, pp 85.

Kappel, L.C. and Zidenberg, S. (1999). Manganese: Present Knowledge in nutrition. In: Brown ML (Ed.), International Life Sciences Institute Nutrition Foundation, Washington. pp. 308.

Kaur, H. and Arora, S. P. (1995). Dietary effects on ruminant livestock reproduction with particular reference to protein. *Nutrition Research Reviews,* **8:** 121-136.

Kellogg, D.W. (1990). Zinc methionine affects performance of lactating cows. *Feedstuffs,* **62**: 35.

Kessy, B.M. and Noakes, D.E. (1979). The use of the starch grain and phenolsulphophthalein test to investigate infertile cows. *Vet. Rec.,* **105**: 489-491.

Khilare, K.P. (2007). Trace minerals and reproduction in animals. *Intas Polivet,* **8**(2): 308-314.

Kimura, M. T.; T. Nakao; M. Moriyoshi and K. Kawata. (1987). Luteal phase deficiency as a possible cause of repeat breeding in dairy cows. *Br. Vet. J.* **143**: 560.

Kirsz, K. and Zieba, D. A. (2012). Selected hypothalamic factors integrating reproduction and energy balance control in animals, *Medycyna Weterynaryjna,* **68**(1): 35–39.

Kothari, B. J.; Renton, C. D.; Munro and McFarlane, J. (1978). Use of the Phenol-sulpho-naphthalene dye test foe fallopian tube patency in cattle. *Vet. Record,* **103**: 229-232.

Kumar, A. K.; Dangi, S.S.; Mahla, A.S.; Rajoriya, J.S. and Purohit, G. N. (2012). Role of nitric oxide in animal reproduction. *Theriogenol Insight,* **2**: 137-144.

Kumar, S. and Agarwal, S. K. (1986): Studies on ovarian dysfunction in rural bovines. *The Indian Vet. Med. J.,* **10**: 125-126.

Kumar, S.; Agarwal, S. K. and Purbey, L. N. (1988): Reproductive disorders in non-descript rural buffaloes. *The Indian Vet. Med. J.,* **12**: 125-126.

Kumar, S.; Pandey, A.K.; Ahmed, W.; Razzaque, A. and Dwivedi, D.K. (2011). Importance of micro minerals in reproductive performance of livestock. *Veterinary World,* **4**(5): 230-233.

Lafi, S.Q.; Kaneene, J.B.; Black, J.R. and Lioyd, J.W. (1992). Epidemiological and economic study of the repeat breeder syndrome in Michingan dairy cattle II. Economic modeling. *Prev. Vet. Med.*,**14**: 99-114.

Larson, L. L., and P. J. H. Ball. (1992). Regulation of estrous cycles in dairy cattle: a review. *Theriogenology*, **38**: 255.

Lin, J. H. ; Wu, L. S.; Wu, Y.L.; Lin, C.S.; Yang, N.Y.J. (2002). Aquapuncture Therapy of Repeat Breeding in Dairy Cattle. *Am. J. Chin. Med.*, **30**: 397.

Lindemann, M.D. (1996). Novel use of biotechnology in farm animal nutrition. In : Alltech's European & Southern African Lecture Tour. pp. 35-53.

Lopez, H.; Kanitz, F.D.; Moreira, V.R.; Satter, L.D. and Wiltbank, M.C. (2004). Reproductive performance of dairy cows fed two concentrations of phosphorus. *Journal of Dairy Science*, **87**: 146-157.

Lopez-Gatius, F. (1995). Intraperitoneal insemination in repeat-breeder cows: a preliminary report. *Theriogenology*, **44**: 153-158.

Lucy, M. C. (2001). Reproductive loss in high producing dairy cattle: where will it end? *J. Dairy Sci.* **84**: 1277-1293.

Lyons, T.P. (1993). Bioscience Centres: Forging links between industry and academia. In: "Biotechnology in the Feed Industry", Proc. Alltech's 9th Sym. pp. 1-25.

Mahan, D.C. and Kim, Y.Y. (1995). Effect of inorganic or organic selenium at two dietary levels on reproductive performance and tissue selenium concentrations in first-parity gilts and their progeny. *J. Amin. Sci.* **74**: 2711-2718.

Mann, G. E. and G. E. Lamming. (1995). Progesterone inhibition of the development of the luteolytic signal in cows. *J. Reprod. Fertil.*, **104**: 1-5.

Mattos, R.; Charles, R. S. and Thatcher, W. W. (2000). Effects of dietary fatty acids on reproduction in ruminants. *Reviews of Reproduction*, **5**: 38–45.

Mc Ardle, C.A and A.P. Holtorf. (1989). Oxytocin and progesterone release from bovine corpus luteal cells in culture; Effects of insulin like growth factor I, insulin and prostaglandins. *Endocrinology*, **124**: 1278-1286.

Mc Donald, R.J.; McKay, G.W. and Thomson, J.D. (1961). The use of organic iodine in treatment of repeat breeder cows. *In:* Proceeding of the IVth International Congress on Animal Reproduction, pp. 679-681.

Mehta, G. B.; Bhavsar, B. K. and Kodagali, S. B. (1986). Ovulatory disturbances in repeat breeding crossbred cattle. *Indian J. Anim. Reprod.*,**7**(2): 63-65.

Mitiku, T.; Ramaswamy, V.; Chanie, M. and Fentahun, T. (2012). Commonness of Reiterate Breeder in Dairy Cattle in Gondar, Ethiopia. *Advances in Biological Research,* **6**(6): 226-230.

Modi, L.C.; Patel, P.A.; Patel, S.P.; Patel, G.G.; Joshi, A.H. and Suthar, D.N. (2011). Prevalence of reproductive problems in Mehsana milk shed area of Gujarat. *Int. J. Anim. Vet. Med. Sci.,* **5**: 424-428.

National Research Council (NRC) (2001). In: Nutrients requirement of dairy cattle, 7th rev. ed. Natl. Acad. Sci, Washington D.C.

Neglia, G.; Restucci, B.; Russo, M.; Vecchio, D.; Gasparrini, B. and Prandi, A. (2015). Early development and function of the corpus luteum and relationship to pregnancy in buffalo. *Theriogenology,* **83**: 959-967.

Nishany, K.B.M.; Ramachandra, M.B.P.; Mahipala, K.; Jayawardane, V.P. and Wijayagunawardane, M.P.B. (2013). Influence of energy balance on reproductive performance and milk production of dairy cows at pre-partum and early lactation periods. *International Journal of Animal and Veterinary Advances,* **5**: 98-102.

Nix, K.J.; Roberts, S. and Wiltbank, J.N. (1981). Using short-term calf removal and flushing to improve pregnancy rate. In: Beef Cattle Research in Texas. Texas Agricultural Experiment Station. pp. 60-68

Noakes, D. E.; Parkinson, T.J. and England, G.C. W. (2001). In: Arthur's Veterinary Reproduction and Obstetrics. Harcourt (India) Private Limited, New Delhi-110048.

NRC. (2001). Nutrient Requirements of Dairy Cattle: Seventh Revised Edition. National Research Council, National Academy of Sciences. Washington, D.C.

Ocon, O. M., and Hansen, P. J. (2003). Disruption of bovine oocytes and preimplantation embryos by urea and acidic pH. *J. Dairy Sci.,* **86**: 1194-1200.

Parmer, K. I.; V. M. Mehta and J. M. Patel. (1986). Biochemical profile in repeat breeding crossbred cows relations to different phases of oestrous cycle. *Indian. J. Anim. Reprod.,* **2**: 31-35.

Patterson, H.H.; Adams, D.C.; Klopfenstein, T.J.; Clark, R.T. and Teichert, B. (2003). Supplementation to meet metabolizable protein requirements of primiparous beef heifers: II. Pregnancy and Economics. *J. Anim. Sci.*, **81**: 503-570.

Peñagaricano, F.; Souza, A.H.; Carvalho, P.D.; Driver, A.M.; Gambra, R.; Kropp, J.; Hackbart, K.S.; Luchini, D.; Shaver, R.D.; Wiltbank, M.C. and Khatib, H. (2013). Effect of maternal methionine supplementation on the transcriptome of bovine preimplantation embryos. *In*: PLoS One 8:e72302.

Perez-Marin, C.C. and Espana, F. (2007). Estrus expression and ovarian function in repeat breeder cows,monitored by ultrasonography and progesterone assay. *Reprod. Dom. Anim.*, **42**: 449-456.

Pierson, R.A. and Ginther, O.J. (1984). Ultrasonography of the bovine ovary. *Theriogenology*, **21**: 495-504.

Pirestani, A. and Maybodi, A.E. (2015). Effect of Diet Energy on Some Reproduction Indices and Hormones at Different Phase of Estrus Cycle in Holstein Heifers. *International Journal of Life Sciences Biotechnology and Pharma Research*, **4**(2): 123-34.

Pradhan, R. and Nakaghosi, N. (2003). Reproductive Disorder in Cattle due to Nutritional Status. *Journal of International Development and Cooperation*, **14**(1): 45-66.

Prasad, A.S. (1979). Clinical, biochemical and pharmacological role of zinc. *Ann. Rev. Pharmacol. Toxicol.*, **19**: 393.

Prohaska, J.R. and Lukasewycz, O.A. (1990). Effect of copper deficiency on the immune system. In : Nutrients and immune functions (A. Bendich, M. Phillips & R.P. Tengerdy, eds). *Adv. Exp. Med. Biol.*, **262**: 123, Plenum Press, New York.

Purohit, G.N. (2008). Recent development of in the diagnosis and therapy of repeat breeding cows and buffaloes. *CAB Reviews: Perspectives in Agriculture, Veterinary Science, Nutrition and Natural Resources*, **3**(62): 1-33.

Purohit, G.N.; Ruhil, S.; Chaudhary, A.K.; Chaudhary, V.; Gaur, M. and Jeenger, K. (2013). Hysteroscopic visualization of bubaline uterus. *Theriogenol Insight* , **3**: 67-70.

Pursley, J.R.; Kosorok, M.R. and Wiltbank, M.C. (1997a). Reproductive management of lactating dairy cows using synchronization of ovulation. *J Dairy Sci*, **80**: 301-306.

Pursley, J.R.; Mee, M.O. and Wiltbank, M.C. (1995). Synchronization of ovulation in dairy cows using $PGF_2\alpha$ and GnRH. *Theriogenology* , **44**: 915-923.

Pursley, J.R.; Wiltbank, M.C.; Stevenson, J.S.; Ottobre, J.S.; Garverick, H.A.; Anderson, L.L. (1997b). Pregnancy rates per artificial insemination for cows and heifers inseminated at a synchronized ovulation or synchronized estrus. *J Dairy Sci,* **80**: 295-300.

Rahbar, B.; Safdar, A. H. A. and Kor, N. M. (2014). Mechanisms through which fat supplementation could enhance reproduction in farm animal. *European Journal of Experimental Biology,* **4**(1): 340-348.

Rajamahendran, R. (1994). Clinical and research applications of real-time ultrasonography in bovine reproduction: A review. *Can. Vet. J.,* **35**: 563-572.

Rajkumar, R. and Durairajan, R. (2016). Effect of Co synch method of synchronization on fertility in repeat breeding cows. *In*: Compendium, XXXII Annual convention of ISSAR, pp. 54.

Randhawa, S.S. and Randhawa, C.S. (1994). Trace element imbalances as a cause of infertility in farm animals. Recent advances in Animal Reproduction and Gynaecology. In: Proceedings of the summer institute, held at PAU, Ludhiana on 25th July to 13th August, 1994, pp. 103-121.

Reeves, J.J.; Rantanen, N.W. and Hauser, M. (1984). Transrectal real-time ultrasound scanning of the cow reproductive tract. *Theriogenology,* **21**: 485-494.

Rhoads, M. L.; Rhoads, R. P.; Gilbert, R. O.; Toole, R. and Butler, W. R. (2006). Detrimental effects of high plasma urea nitrogen levels on viability of embryos from lactating dairy cows. *Anim. Reprod. Sci.,* **91**: 1-10.

Richards, M. W.; R. P. Wettemann and M. H. Schenemann. (1989). Nutitional anestrus in beef cows: Concentrations of glucose and nonestrified fatty acids in plasma and insulin in serum. *J. Anim. Sci.,* **67**: 2354-2362.

Roberts, S.J. (1971). Veterinary Obstetrics and Genital Diseases (Theriogenology). Edited by S.J. Roberts, 2nd Ed. 1971. pp. 421, 433, 376, 353-357, 378, 501.

Robinson, J. J.; Ashworth, C.J.; Tom, J.R. and Mcevoy, G. (2006). Nutrition and fertility in ruminant livestock. *Animal Feed Science and Technology,* **126**(3): 259-276.

Rodney, R.M.; Celi, P.; Scott, W.; Breinhild, K. and Lean, I. J. (2015). Effects of dietary fat on fertility of dairy cattle: A meta-analysis and meta-regression. *J. Dairy Sci,* **98**: 5601–5620.

Royal, M.D.; G.E. Mann and A.P.F. Flint. (2000). Strategies for reversing the trend towards subfertility in dairy cattle. *Vet. J.* **160**: 53-60.

Ryan, D. P.; Spoon, R. A.; Griffith, M. K. and Williams, G. L. (1994). Ovarian follicular recruitment, granulosa cell steroidogenic potential and growth hormone/insulin-like growth factor-1 relationships in suckled beef cows consuming high lipid diets: Effects of graded differences in body condition maintained during the puerperium. *Domest. Anim. Endocrinol*, **11**: 161-174.

Ryan, D. P.; Spoon, R. A.; Griffith, M. K. and Williams, G. L. (2014). Recruitment, granulosa cell steroidogenic potential and growth hormone/insulin-like growth factor-1 relationships in suckled beef cows consuming high lipid diets: Effects of reproduction in lactating dairy cows. *Advances in Dairy Technology*, **12**: 213-232.

Sah, S.K. and Nakao, T. (2006). Characteristics of repeat breeding buffaloes in Nepal. *J. Reprod. Dev.*, **52**: 335-341.

Santana, A.O.; Oba, E.; Langoni, H. and Uribe-Velasquez, L.F. (1998). *In:* Avalia_ao bacteriologica do endometrio em femeas bovinas repetidoras de cio. *Arch Reprod. Ani.*, **6**: 62-71.

Saxena, M. S. (2004). Repat breeding in cows and buffaloes. *In:* Proceding of National symposium on conservation and propagation of indigenous breeds of cattle and buffaloes, Uttaranchal. Pp 26-28.

Schalm, O. W.; Carrol, J. E. and Jain, N. C. (1971). Bovine Mastitis. 1st Ed. Lea and Febiger, Philadelphia, USA. pp. 132-153.

Schweigert, F.J. and Zucker, H. (1988). Concentration of vitamin A , beta-carotene and vitamin E in individual bovine follicles of different quality. *Journal of Reproduction and Fertility*, **82**: 575-579.

Shaham-Albalancy, A., Folman, Y., Kaim, M., Rosenberg, M. and Wolfenson, D. (2001). Delayed effect of low progesterone concentrations on bovine uterine PGF(2alpha) secretion in the subsequent oestrous cycle. *J. Reproduction*, **122**: 643-648.

Shahneh, A.Z.; Mohammadi, Z.; Fazeli, H.; Babak, M.H. and Dirandeh, E. (2008). The effect of GnRH injection on plasma progesterone concentrations, conception rate and ovulation rate in Iranian Holstein cows. *J. Anim. Vet. Adv.* **7**(9): 1137-1141.

Sheldon, I. M.; Lewis, G. S.; Le Blanc, S. and Gilbert, R. O. (2006). Defining postpartum uterine disease in cattle. *Theriogenology*, **65**(8): 1516-1530.

Shiraz khan; A. Thangavel and S. Selvasubramaniyan. (2010). Blood Biochemical profile in repeat Breeding cows. *Tamilnadu J. Veterinary & Animal Sciences,* **6**(2): 75-80.

Short, R.E. and Adams, D.C.(1988). Nutritional and hormonal interrelationships in beef cattle reproduction. *Canadian Journal of Animal Science,* **68**: 29-39.

Shrestha, H. K.; Nakao, T.; Higaki, T.; Suzuki, T. and Akita, M. (2004). Resumption of postpartum ovarian cyclicity in high-producing Holstein cows. *Theriogenology,* **61**(4): 637-49.

Sinclair, K.D.; Garnsworthy, P.C.; Mann, G.E. and Sinclair, L.A. (2014). Reducing dietary protein in dairy cow diets: implications for nitrogen utilization, milk production, welfare and fertility. *Animal,* **8**: 262-274.

Singh, B.; Fernando, S.; Renee, B. and Heriberto, R. (2005). Pregnancy rates in Repeat-breeder heifers following multiple Artificial Inseminations during spontaneous oestrus. *Acta Veterinaria Scandinavica,* **46:** 1-12.

Singh, J.; Dadarwal, D.; Honparkhe, M. and Kumar, A. (2009). Incidences of various etiological factors responsible for repeat breeding syndrome in cattle and buffaloes. *Int. J. Vet. Med.* **6**(1): 26-30.

Sreenan, J. M.; M. G. Diskin and L. Dunne. (1996). Embryonic mortality: the major cause of reproductive wastage in cattle. *In:* Proc. 47th Annual Meeting Europ. Assoc. Anim. Prod., Lillehammer.

Staats, D.A.; Lohr, D.P. and Colby, H.D. (1988). Effects of tocopherol depletion on the regional differences in adrenal microsomal lipid peroxidation and steroid metabolism. *Endocrinology,* **23**: 975-980.

Stener-Victorin, E.; Waldenstrom, U. and Andersson, S.A. (1996). Reductio of blood flow impedance in the uterine arteries of infertile women with electro-acupuncture. *Hum. Reprod.,* **11**(6): 1314-1317.

Stevenson, J. S. and M. O. Mee. (1990). Pregnancy rates of Holstein cows after postinsemination treatment with a progesterone-releasing intravaginal device. *J. Dairy Sci.,* **74**: 3849-3856.

Stevenson, J.S.; Call, E.P.; Scoby, R.K. and Phatak, A.P. (1990). Double insemination and gonadotropin releasing hormone treatment of repeat-breeding dairy cattle. *J dairy Sc.,***73**: 1766-1772.

Stock, A. E. and Fortune, J. E. (1993). Ovarian follicular dominance in cattle: relationship betweenprolonged growth of the ovulatory follicle and endocrine parameters. *Endocrinology,* **132**: 1108-1114.

Talukdar D. (2016). *In:* Ovulation induction techniques and its therapeutic efficacy in cattle. Lambart Academic Publishing (LAP), Germany.

Talukdar, D. J.; Ahmed, K.; Deori, S. and Talukdar, P. (2016). Repeat breeding syndrome in dairy cows: influence of various etiological factors. *The North- East Veterinarian,* **XVI**(3): 30-32.

Talukdar, D. J.; Shyam, J.; Talukdar, P.; Ahmed, K. and Gogoi, R. (2015). Documentation of traditional herbal medicines for reproductive disorders of livestock in Kamrup District of Assam. *International Journal of Agricultural Science and Research,* **5**(6): 221-228.

Talukdar, D. J.; Nath, K. C.; Bonia, K. K. and Deori, S. (2015). Cyclic changes in blood biochemical profiles following induction of ovulation in anovulatory crossbred cows. *The North- East Veterinarian,* **XV**(1): 22-24.

Talukdar, D. J.; Nath, K.C.; Dutta, J. and Talukdar, P. (2013). Therapeutic efficacy of hCG and manual pressure in the management of anovulation in cattle. *The Indian J. Field Veterinarians,* **8**(4): 7-10.

Talukdar, D.J. (2010). Induction of ovulation in repeat breeder crossbred cattle with hCG and manual pressure. M.V.Sc. Thesis, Assam Agricultural University, Guwahati, Assam, India.

Tamminga, S. (2006). The effect of the supply of rumen degradable protein and metabolisable protein on negative energy balance and fertility in dairy cows. *Anim. Reprod. Sci.,* **96**: 227-239.

Tanaka, H.; Hishinuma, M.; Takahashi, Y. and Kanagawa, H. (1994). Developmental competence of oocytes from the ovaries of repeat-breeding cows after in vitro fertlization. *J. Vet. Med. Sci.,* **56**(3): 547-548.

Tandle, M.K. and Purohit, G.N. (2013). Genital tract affections in the buffalo. *In:* Purohit G.N., editor. *Bubaline theriogenology.* Ithaca NY: International Veterinary Information Service; NY.

Thatcher, M. M.; C. R. Staples; G. Desnoyers; D. Oldick and E. P. Shmitt. (1994). Embryo health and mortility in sheep and cattle. *J. Anim. Sci.* **72**(3): 16.

Thatcher, W. W. and C. R. Staples. (2000). Effects of dietary fat supplementation on reproduction in lactating dairy cows. *Advances in Dairy Technology,* **12**: 213-232.

Thatcher, W.; Santos, J. E. and Staples, C. R. (2011). Dietary manipulations to improve embryonic survival in cattle. *Theriogenology,* **76**: 1619-1631.

Tuormaa, T.E. (2000). Chromium, Selenium, Copper and other trace minerals in health and reproduction. *J. Orthomolecular medicine*, **15**: 145-157.

Underwood, E.J. (1981). In: The mineral nutrition of livestock, pp.88-94, CAB International, London, England.

Vijayarajan, A.; Jayaganthan, P.; Prabaharan, V.; Rajkumar, R.; Sivakumar, A. and Raja, S. (2016). Effect of Ovsynch plus CIDR protocol in management of repeat breeding crossbred Jersey cows. *In*: Compendium, XXXII Annual convention of ISSAR, pp. 44.

Vohra, S.C.; C.V. Dindorkar and A.S. Kaikini. (1995). Studies on blood serum levels of certain biochemical constituents in normal cycling and anestrous cross bred cows. *Indian J. Anim. Reprod.*, **16**: 85-87.

Waldmann, A.; Reksen, O.; Landsverk, K.; Ropstad, E.; Kommisrud, E.; Dahl, E. and Refdal, A.O. (2000). Progesterone at first insemination-effects on non-return and repeat-breeding. *In:* 14th International Congress on Animal Reproduction, Stockholm, pp. 87.

Wang, J.Y.; Owen, F.G. and Larson, L.L. (1988). Effect of beta-carotene supplementation on reproductive performance of lactating Holstein cows. *J. Dairy Sci.*, **71**: 181-186.

Wathes, D. C.; Fenwick, M.; Cheng, Z.; Bourne, N.; Llewellyn, S. and Morris, D. G. (2007). Influence of negative energy balance on cyclicity and fertility in the high producing dairy cows. *Theriogenology*, **68**: 232-241.

Whiteside, W. H. (1939). Observation on a new test for the presence of mastitis in milk. *Canad. Publ. healt. J.* **30**: 40.

Wichtell, J.J.; Craigie, A.L.; Thompson, K.G. and William, N.B. (1996). Effect of selenium and A-tocopherol supplementation on postpartum reproductive function of dairy heifers at pasture. *Theriogenology*, **46**: 491-502.

Willard, S. S.; Gandy, S.; Bowers, K.; Graves, A.; Elias and C. Whisnant. (2003). The effects of GnRH administration post insemination on serum concentrations of progesterone and pregnancy rates in dairy cattle exposed to mild summer heat stress. *Theriogenology*, **59**: 1799-1810.

Wiltbank, M.C.; Garcia-Guerra, A.; Carvalho, P.D.; Hackbart, K.S.; Bender, R.W.; Souza, A.H.; Toledo, M.Z.; Baez, G.M.; Surjus, R.S. and Sartori, R. (2014). Effects of energy and protein nutrition in the dam on embryonic development. *Anim. Reprod.*, **11**(3): 168-182.

Wiltbank, M.C.; Souza, A.H.; Carvalho, P.A.; Cunha, A.P.; Giordano, J.O.; Fricke, P.M.; Baez, G.M. and Diskin, M.G. (2014). Physiological and practical effects of progesterone on reproduction in dairy cattle. *Animal*, **8**(1): 70-81.

Wiltbank, M.C.; Weigel, K.A. and Caraviello, D.Z. (2007). Recent studies on nutritional factors affecting reproductive efficiency in U.S. dairy herds. In: Western Dairy Management Conference, New York, pp. 78-82.

Y. B. Grohan, H. Erb and H. Saoloemi. (1995). Epidemiology of reproductive disorders in dairy cattle. *J. Prev. Med.*, **8**: 25-39.

Yasothai, R. (2014). Importance of protein on reproduction in dairy cattle. *International Journal of Science Environment and Technology*, **3**(6): 2081–2083.

Yeager, A.E.; Mohammed, M.O.; Meyers Wallen, V.N.; Vannerson, L. and Concannon, P.W. (1992). Utrasonographic appearance of the uterus, placenta, fetus and fetal membranes throughout accurately timed pregnancy in beagles. *Am. J. Vet. Res.*, **53**: 342-351.

Yildiz, H.; Kaygusuzoglu, E.; Kaya1, M. and Cenesiz, M. (2009). Effect of post-mating GnRH treatment on serum progesterone, luteinizing hormone levels, duration of estrous cycle and pregnancy rates in cows. *Pakistan Vet. J.*, **29**(3): 110-114.

Youngquist, R.S. and Threlfall, W.R. (2007). *In:* Current Therapy in Large Animal Theriogenology.2nd Edition. Published by the author. Distributed by Saunders, St. Louis, Missouri. pp 442.

Yu, O.H. and Tak-yin, M. H. (1993). The efficiency of Povidone iodine pessaries in a start, low-dose treatment regime on candidal, trichomonal and nonspecific vaginitis. *Posgrad. Med. J.*, **69**(3): 58-61.

□□□

Index

❑❑❑

About the Authors

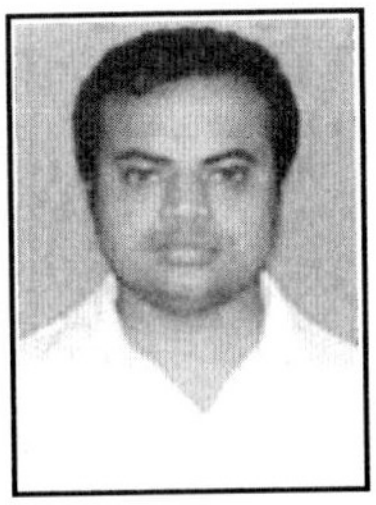

Dibyajyoti Talukdar was born on 22nd July, 1983 in Kamrup district of Assam. He has earned B.V.Sc. & A.H. degree from Assam Agricultural University, Jorhat. After graduation he worked as a Veterinary consultant for the period of three years at Gana Satirtha Manch, Human Resourse Development Organisation, N.G.O. He has completed his M.V.Sc. degree with distinction in the year 2010 from Assam Agricultural University, Jorhat in the discipline Animal Reproduction, Gynaecology & Obstetrics. He worked as a Research Associate at ICAR MSP on Pig, AAU, Khanapara for the period of one year. After that he joined doctoral progrmme in the year 2011 and he completed his Ph D degree in the discipline Animal Reproduction, Gynaecology & Obstetrics from Assam Agricultural University, Jorhat with distinction in the year 2014. He has completed ICAR-NET in the discipline Animal Reproduction, Gynaecology & Obstetrics. After completing Ph D degree, he worked as a Project Scientist at Mugagen Laboratories Pvt. Ltd., IIT Guwahati for the period of one year. Presently he is working as a Teaching Associate at Department of Animal Reproduction, Gynaecology & Obstetrics, College of Veterinary Sciences & Animal Husbandry, Central Agricultural University, Selesih, Aizawl, Mizoram, India. He has published one book, twenty six research articles at different national and international journals, two manuals and several popular articles and folder. He has attended many national and international seminars, symposium and refresher training courses. Now- a-days he is actively involved in teaching, research and extension activities at College of Veterinary Sciences & Animal Husbandry, Central Agricultural University, Selesih, Aizawl, Mizoram, India.

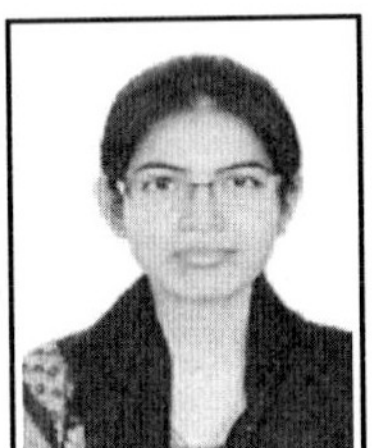

Papori Talukdar was born on 22nd April, 1986 in Kamrup district of Assam. She has earned B.V.Sc. & A.H. degree from Assam Agricultural University, Jorhat. After graduation she joined master degree programme and she completed her M.V.Sc. degree with distinction in the year 2012 from Assam Agricultural University, Jorhat in the discipline Animal Nutrition. She has completed ICAR-NET in the discipline Animal Nutrition. She worked as a Project Assistant at ICAR NRC on Pig, Guwahati for the period of six months. After that she joined doctoral progrmme in the year 2012 at NDRI, Karnal and she completed her Ph D degree in the year 2016 in the discipline Dairy Cattle Nutrition. After completing Ph D degree, she joined as an Assistant Professor, Department of Animal Nutrition, Khalsa College of Veterinary & Animal Sciences, Amritsar, Punjab, India. She has published one book, one book chapter, twelve research articles at different national and international journals, and several popular articles and folder. She has attended many national and international seminars, symposium and refresher training courses. Now- a-days she is actively involved in teaching, research and extension activities at Khalsa College of Veterinary & Animal Sciences, Amritsar, Punjab.